300
Full-Body Body Weight Workouts Book for Men and Women

300
Full-Body Body Weight Workouts Book for Men and Women

Big Guide to 300 Bodyweight Exercises with Step-by-Step Guides, Images, and Muscle Targeting Information for Muscle Building & Fat Loss

Be.Bull Publishing Group

Authors:

Be.Bull Publishing Group

Mauricio Vasquez

First Printing: August 2024

ISBN-978-1-998402-63-2 (Paperback)

ISBN-978-1-998402-64-9 (Hardcover)

TIPS

- Adjust the number of repetitions and the time cap for the workouts according to your capabilities, skills and physical condition
- Listen to your body and don't push yourself too hard
- If you don't have enough space where to run, you can do jumping jacks. 100-meter run is approximately equivalent to 50 jumping jacks
- Walk into the gym with a workout already selected for you
- Get motivated with a fun workout playlist
- Put your phone on airplane mode
- Start your workout with some stretches
- Log the details of each workout so you can track your progress. You can track time and number of repetitions
- Enjoy your workouts

Dear valued customer,

Your opinion matters!

By leaving a review using the QR code provided, you can help fellow readers discover and enjoy this book. Your feedback will guide others in making informed decisions and enhance their reading experience.

Thank you for contributing to our reading community!

Mauricio

Disclaimer

1. Be.Bull Publishing (Aria Capri International Inc.) strongly recommends that you consult with your physician before beginning any exercise program or workout. You should be in good physical condition and be able to participate in the exercises and workouts. We are not a licensed medical care provider and represents that we have no expertise in diagnosing, examining, or treating medical conditions of any kind, or in determining the effect of any specific exercise or workout on a medical condition.

2. You should understand that when participating in any exercise or workout, there is the possibility of physical injury. If you engage in the exercises and workouts of this book, you agree that you do so at your own risk, are voluntarily participating in these activities, assume all risk of injury to yourself, and agree to release and discharge Be.Bull Publishing (Aria Capri International Inc.) from any and all claims or causes of action, known or unknown, arising out of this book and videos.

3. The information provided through this book is not intended to be a substitute for professional medical advice, diagnosis or treatment. Never disregard professional medical advice, or delay in seeking it, because of something you have read on this book or watch in the videos. Never rely on information on this book or videos in place of seeking professional medical advice.

4. Be.Bull Publishing (Aria Capri International Inc.) is not responsible or liable for any advice, course of treatment, diagnosis or any other information, services or products that you obtain through this book or videos. You are encouraged to consult with your doctor with regard to the information contained on or through this book or videos. After reading this book or watching videos from this book, you are encouraged to review the information carefully with your professional healthcare provider.

FREE DOWNLOAD

BONUS No 1 - 1000 Full-Body Workouts

To access extra 1,000 workouts to stay motivated and avoid workout boredom with endless variety, scan this QR code:

BONUS No 2- Logging Sheets of Your Workout Book

To access your free e-copy of this workout book, scan this QR code:

If you want to add more variety to your workouts, scan this QR code to check these workout books!

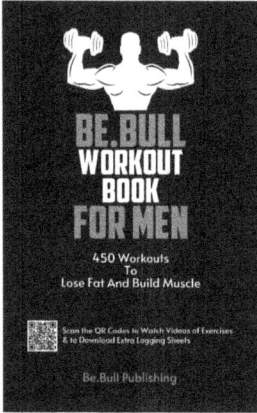

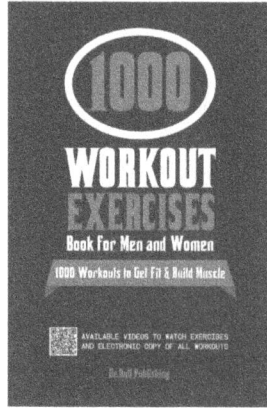

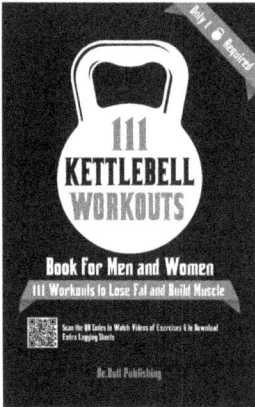

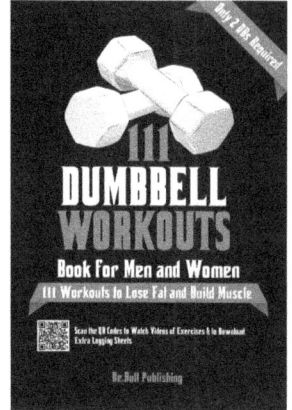

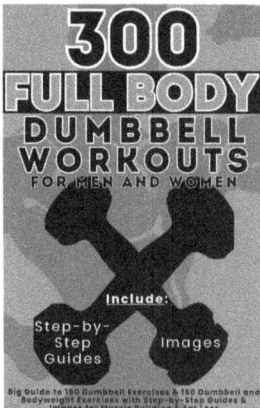

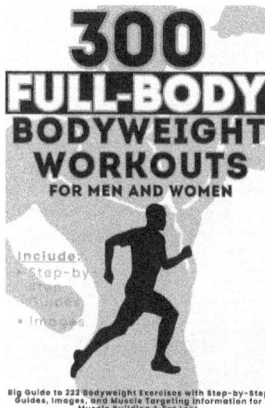

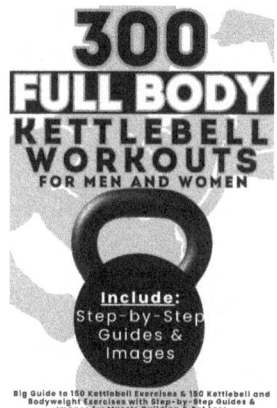

Workout No.	Workout	Main Muscle Groups	Instructions
1	**5 Rounds for time:**		
	(1) 10 Burpees	Full Body, Core, Legs	Perform a jump, squat, kick back into a push-up, return up. Repeat quickly.
	(2) 15 Push Ups	Chest, Shoulders, Triceps	Lower body to ground, push up with arms.
	(3) 20 Air Squats	Legs, Glutes, Core	Stand, bend knees to lower body, keep back straight.
2	**As many rounds as possible in 20 mins:**		
	(1) 10 Pull-Ups	Back, Biceps, Core	Pull body up on bar, chin above hands.
	(2) 20 Walking Lunges	Legs, Glutes, Core	Step forward into a lunge, move forward alternating legs.
	(3) 30 Sit-Ups	Core, Hip Flexors, Abdominals	Lift shoulders off ground, contract abdominals.
3	**4 Rounds for time:**		
	(1) 15 Box Jumps	Legs, Glutes, Calves	Jump onto and off a box repeatedly, land softly.
	(2) 20 Push-Ups	Chest, Shoulders, Triceps	Lower body to ground, push up with arms.
	(3) 25 Jumping Jacks	Full Body, Cardio, Calves	Jump to spread legs and clap hands overhead.
4	**Every minute on the minute for 10 mins:**		
	(1) 10 Burpees	Full Body, Core, Legs	Perform a jump, squat, kick back into a push-up, return up. Repeat quickly.
	(2) 15 Air Squats	Legs, Glutes, Core	Stand, bend knees to lower body, keep back straight.
5	**21-15-9 Reps of:**		
	(1) Push-Ups	Chest, Shoulders, Triceps	Lower body to ground, push up with arms.
	(2) Sit-Ups	Core, Hip Flexors, Abdominals	Lift shoulders off ground, contract abdominals.
	(3) Air Squats	Legs, Glutes, Core	Stand, bend knees to lower body, keep back straight.
6	**45 seconds work, 15 seconds rest, 5 rounds:**		
	(2) High Knees	Legs, Cardio, Core	Run in place lifting knees high, maintain pace.
	(3) Mountain Climbers	Core, Shoulders, Cardio	Run in place in plank position, drive knees to chest.
	(4) Jumping Jacks	Full Body, Cardio, Calves	Jump to spread legs and clap hands overhead.
7	**40 seconds work, 20 seconds rest, 4 rounds:**		
	(1) Burpees	Full Body, Core, Legs	Perform a jump, squat, kick back into a push-up, return up. Repeat quickly.
	(2) Bicycle Crunches	Core, Obliques, Abdominals	Lie down, alternate elbows to opposite knees cycling legs.
	(3) Plank	Core, Shoulders, Abdominals	Hold body straight on elbows, maintain line.

Workout No.	Workout	Main Muscle Groups	Instructions
8	**50 seconds work, 10 seconds rest, 8 rounds:**		
	(1) Jump Squats	Legs, Glutes, Core	Jump from squat position, land softly. Repeat quickly.
	(2) Push-Ups	Chest, Shoulders, Triceps	Lower body to ground, push up with arms.
	(3) Flutter Kicks	Core, Hip Flexors, Abdominals	Lie on back, alternately kick legs in small, rapid motion.
9	**45 seconds work, 15 seconds rest, 4 rounds:**		
	(1) Skater Squats	Legs, Glutes, Core	Balance on one leg, squat, touch opposite hand to foot.
	(2) Tricep Dips	Triceps, Shoulders, Chest	Dip body between bars, focus on triceps.
	(3) Russian Twists	Core, Obliques, Abdominals	Twist torso holding weight, seated on ground.
10	**40 seconds work, 20 seconds rest, 5 rounds:**		
	(1) Burpees	Full Body, Core, Legs	Perform a jump, squat, kick back into a push-up, return up. Repeat quickly.
	(2) Jumping Jacks	Full Body, Cardio, Calves	Jump to spread legs and clap hands overhead.
	(3) Plank Rotation	Core, Shoulders, Obliques	Rotate body in plank, extend arm upward, switch sides.
11	**As many rounds as possible in 10 mins of:**		
	(1) Burpees (10 reps)	Full Body, Core, Legs	Jump, squat down, kick back into a push-up, return up. Perform 10 reps.
	(2) Side Plank (30 seconds each side)	Core, Shoulders, Obliques	Support body on one arm, side facing ground. Hold for 30 seconds each side.
	(3) Bear Crawl (20 meters)	Full Body, Core, Shoulders	Crawl forward on all fours, hips down, move quickly. Perform 20 meters.
12	**45 seconds work, 15 seconds rest per exercise for 4 rounds:**		
	(1) High Knees	Legs, Core, Cardio	Run in place lifting knees high, maintain pace. Perform for 45 seconds.
	(2) Bicycle Crunches	Core, Obliques, Hip Flexors	Lie down, alternate elbows to opposite knees cycling legs. Perform for 45 seconds.
	(3) Jumping Jacks	Full Body, Cardio, Legs	Jump to spread legs and clap hands overhead. Perform for 45 seconds.
	Push-Up w/ Extension	Chest, Shoulders, Core	Perform push-up, extend one arm forward, alternate. Perform for 45 seconds.
13	**Every minute on the minute for 20 mins:**		
	(1) Pull-Ups (5 reps)	Back, Biceps, Shoulders	Pull body up on bar, chin above hands. Perform 5 reps.
	(2) Glute Bridge (10 reps)	Glutes, Core, Hamstrings	Lift hips while lying on back, feet flat on ground. Perform 10 reps.
	(3) Crab Walk (20 meters)	Triceps, Core, Glutes	Walk backward on hands and feet, hips elevated. Perform 20 meters.
14	**As many rounds as possible in 12 mins:**		
	(1) Tuck Jumps (10 reps)	Legs, Core, Cardio	Jump high, tuck knees to chest mid-air. Perform 10 reps.
	(2) Fire Hydrant (15 reps each leg)	Glutes, Core, Hip Flexors	On hands and knees, lift leg to side, keep knee bent. Perform 15 reps each leg.
	(3) Plank Rotation (10 reps each side)	Core, Shoulders, Obliques	Rotate body in plank, extend arm upward, switch sides. Perform 10 reps each side.

Workout No.	Workout	Main Muscle Groups	Instructions
15	**5 Rounds for time:**		
	(1) Inchworm (10 reps)	Full Body, Core, Shoulders	Walk hands forward from standing, hold plank, walk back. Perform 10 reps.
	(2) Single Leg Squat (10 reps each leg)	Quads, Glutes, Core	Stand on one leg, squat, maintain balance. Perform 10 reps each leg.
	(3) Superman (15 reps)	Lower Back, Glutes, Shoulders	Extend arms and legs while face down, hold position. Perform 15 reps.
16	**40 seconds work, 20 seconds rest per exercise for 4 rounds:**		
	(1) Mountain Climbers	Core, Legs, Shoulders	Run in place in plank position, drive knees to chest. Perform for 45 seconds.
	(2) Flutter Kicks	Core, Hip Flexors, Lower Abs	Lie on back, alternately kick legs in small, rapid motion. Perform for 45 seconds.
	(3) Calf Raises	Calves, Core, Balance	Lift heels off ground, balance on toes, lower slowly. Perform for 45 seconds.
	(4) Side Lunge	Legs, Glutes, Core	Step to side into lunge, keep other leg straight. Perform for 45 seconds.
17	**As many rounds as possible in 10 mins of:**		
	(1) Burpees (10 reps)	Full Body, Core, Legs	Jump, squat down, kick back into a push-up, return up. Perform 10 reps.
	(2) Side Plank (30 seconds each side)	Core, Shoulders, Obliques	Support body on one arm, side facing ground. Hold for 30 seconds each side.
	(3) Bear Crawl (20 meters)	Full Body, Core, Shoulders	Crawl forward on all fours, hips down, move quickly. Perform 20 meters.
18	**As many rounds as possible in 12 mins:**		
	(1) Tuck Jumps (10 reps)	Legs, Core, Cardio	Jump high, tuck knees to chest mid-air. Perform 10 reps.
	(2) Fire Hydrant (15 reps each leg)	Glutes, Core, Hip Flexors	On hands and knees, lift leg to side, keep knee bent. Perform 15 reps each leg.
	(3) Plank Rotation (10 reps each side)	Core, Shoulders, Obliques	Rotate body in plank, extend arm upward, switch sides. Perform 10 reps each side.
19	**Every minute on the minute for 20 mins:**		
	(1) Pull-Ups (5 reps)	Back, Biceps, Shoulders	Pull body up on bar, chin above hands. Perform 5 reps.
	(2) Glute Bridge (10 reps)	Glutes, Core, Hamstrings	Lift hips while lying on back, feet flat on ground. Perform 10 reps.
	(3) Crab Walk (20 meters)	Triceps, Core, Glutes	Walk backward on hands and feet, hips elevated. Perform 20 meters.
20	**30 seconds work, 30 seconds rest per exercise for 4 rounds:**		
	(1) High Knees	Legs, Core, Cardio	Run in place lifting knees high, maintain pace. Perform for 45 seconds.
	(2) Bicycle Crunches	Core, Obliques, Hip Flexors	Lie down, alternate elbows to opposite knees cycling legs. Perform for 45 seconds.
	(3) Jumping Jacks	Full Body, Cardio, Legs	Jump to spread legs and clap hands overhead. Perform for 45 seconds.
	(4) Push-Up w/ Extension	Chest, Shoulders, Core	Perform push-up, extend one arm forward, alternate. Perform for 45 seconds.

Workout No.	Workout		Main Muscle Groups	Instructions
21	**As many rounds as possible in 10 mins of:**			
	(1)	Push-Ups (15 reps)	Chest, Triceps, Shoulders	Lower body to ground, push up with arms. Perform 15 reps.
	(2)	Walking Lunges (20 reps each leg)	Legs, Glutes, Core	Step forward into a lunge, move forward alternating legs. Perform 20 reps each leg.
	(3)	Mountain Climbers (30 seconds)	Core, Legs, Shoulders	Run in place in plank position, drive knees to chest. Perform for 30 seconds.
22	**45 seconds work, 15 seconds rest per exercise for 4 rounds:**			
	(1)	High Knees	Legs, Core, Cardio	Run in place lifting knees high, maintain pace. Perform for 45 seconds.
	(2)	Cross-Body Crunches	Core, Obliques, Hip Flexors	Touch opposite knee to elbow, lying down. Perform for 45 seconds.
	(3)	Jumping Jacks	Full Body, Cardio, Legs	Jump to spread legs and clap hands overhead. Perform for 45 seconds.
	(4)	Fire Hydrants	Glutes, Core, Hip Flexors	On hands and knees, lift leg to side, keep knee bent. Perform for 45 seconds.
23	**Every minute on the minute for 20 mins:**			
	(1)	Pull-Ups (5 reps)	Back, Biceps, Shoulders	Pull body up on bar, chin above hands. Perform 5 reps.
	(2)	Glute Bridge (10 reps)	Glutes, Core, Hamstrings	Lift hips while lying on back, feet flat on ground. Perform 10 reps.
	(3)	Crab Walk (20 meters)	Triceps, Core, Glutes	Walk backward on hands and feet, hips elevated. Perform 20 meters.
24	**As many rounds as possible in 12 mins:**			
	(1)	Tuck Jumps (10 reps)	Legs, Core, Cardio	Jump high, tuck knees to chest mid-air. Perform 10 reps.
	(2)	Fire Hydrant (15 reps each leg)	Glutes, Core, Hip Flexors	On hands and knees, lift leg to side, keep knee bent. Perform 15 reps each leg.
	(3)	Plank Rotation (10 reps each side)	Core, Shoulders, Obliques	Rotate body in plank, extend arm upward, switch sides. Perform 10 reps each side.
25	**5 Rounds for time:**			
	(1)	Inchworm (10 reps)	Full Body, Core, Shoulders	Walk hands forward from standing, hold plank, walk back. Perform 10 reps.
	(2)	Single Leg Squat (10 reps each leg)	Quads, Glutes, Core	Stand on one leg, squat, maintain balance. Perform 10 reps each leg.
	(3)	Superman (15 reps)	Lower Back, Glutes, Shoulders	Extend arms and legs while face down, hold position. Perform 15 reps.
26	**50 seconds work, 10 seconds rest per exercise for 4 rounds:**			
	(1)	Mountain Climbers	Core, Legs, Shoulders	Run in place in plank position, drive knees to chest. Perform for 45 seconds.
	(2)	Flutter Kicks	Core, Hip Flexors, Lower Abs	Lie on back, alternately kick legs in small, rapid motion. Perform for 45 seconds.
	(3)	Calf Raises	Calves, Core, Balance	Lift heels off ground, balance on toes, lower slowly. Perform for 45 seconds.
	(4)	Side Lunge	Legs, Glutes, Core	Step to side into lunge, keep other leg straight. Perform for 45 seconds.

Workout No.	Workout	Main Muscle Groups	Instructions
27	**As many rounds as possible in 10 mins of:**		
	(1) Burpees (10 reps)	Full Body, Core, Legs	Jump, squat down, kick back into a push-up, return up. Perform 10 reps.
	(2) Side Plank (30 seconds each side)	Core, Shoulders, Obliques	Support body on one arm, side facing ground. Hold for 30 seconds each side.
	(3) Bear Crawl (20 meters)	Full Body, Core, Shoulders	Crawl forward on all fours, hips down, move quickly. Perform 20 meters.
28	**As many rounds as possible in 12 mins:**		
	(1) Tuck Jumps (10 reps)	Legs, Core, Cardio	Jump high, tuck knees to chest mid-air. Perform 10 reps.
	(2) Fire Hydrant (15 reps each leg)	Glutes, Core, Hip Flexors	On hands and knees, lift leg to side, keep knee bent. Perform 15 reps each leg.
	(3) Plank Rotation (10 reps each side)	Core, Shoulders, Obliques	Rotate body in plank, extend arm upward, switch sides. Perform 10 reps each side.
29	**Every minute on the minute for 20 mins:**		
	(1) Pull-Ups (5 reps)	Back, Biceps, Shoulders	Pull body up on bar, chin above hands. Perform 5 reps.
	(2) Glute Bridge (10 reps)	Glutes, Core, Hamstrings	Lift hips while lying on back, feet flat on ground. Perform 10 reps.
	(3) Crab Walk (20 meters)	Triceps, Core, Glutes	Walk backward on hands and feet, hips elevated. Perform 20 meters.
30	**45 seconds work, 15 seconds rest per exercise for 4 rounds:**		
	(1) High Knees	Legs, Core, Cardio	Run in place lifting knees high, maintain pace. Perform for 45 seconds.
	(2) Bicycle Crunches	Core, Obliques, Hip Flexors	Lie down, alternate elbows to opposite knees cycling legs. Perform for 45 seconds.
	(3) Jumping Jacks	Full Body, Cardio, Legs	Jump to spread legs and clap hands overhead. Perform for 45 seconds.
	(4) Push-Up w/ Extension	Chest, Shoulders, Core	Perform push-up, extend one arm forward, alternate. Perform for 45 seconds.
31	**As many rounds as possible in 10 mins of:**		
	(1) Box Jumps (15 reps)	Legs, Glutes, Core	Jump onto and off a box repeatedly, land softly. Perform 15 reps.
	(2) Side-to-Side Push-Up (10 reps each side)	Chest, Shoulders, Core	Shift side-to-side during push-ups, engages core. Perform 10 reps each side.
	(3) Windshield Wipers (15 reps)	Core, Obliques, Hip Flexors	Swing legs side-to-side lying down, mimic wiper. Perform 15 reps.
32	**40 seconds work, 20 seconds rest per exercise for 4 rounds:**		
	(1) High Knees	Legs, Core, Cardio	Run in place lifting knees high, maintain pace. Perform for 45 seconds.
	(2) Bear Crawl	Full Body, Core, Shoulders	Crawl forward on all fours, hips down, move quickly. Perform for 45 seconds.
	(3) Flutter Kicks	Core, Hip Flexors, Lower Abs	Lie on back, alternately kick legs in small, rapid motion. Perform for 45 seconds.
	(4) Crab Walk	Triceps, Core, Glutes	Walk backward on hands and feet, hips elevated. Perform for 45 seconds.

Workout No.	Workout	Main Muscle Groups	Instructions
33	**Every minute on the minute for 20 mins:**		
	(1) Pull-Ups (5 reps)	Back, Biceps, Shoulders	Pull body up on bar, chin above hands. Perform 5 reps.
	(2) V-Ups (10 reps)	Core, Hip Flexors, Lower Abs	Lie back, lift legs and torso simultaneously, form 'V'. Perform 10 reps.
	(3) Donkey Kicks (10 reps each leg)	Glutes, Core, Hamstrings	On hands and knees, kick one leg back and up. Perform 10 reps each leg.
34	**As many rounds as possible in 12 mins:**		
	(1) Tuck Jumps (10 reps)	Legs, Core, Cardio	Jump high, tuck knees to chest mid-air. Perform 10 reps.
	(2) Bird Dog (10 reps each side)	Core, Glutes, Shoulders	Extend opposite arm and leg, kneeling position. Perform 10 reps each side.
	(3) Plank (30 seconds)	Core, Shoulders, Back	Hold body straight on elbows, maintain line. Perform for 30 seconds.
35	**5 Rounds for time:**		
	(1) Lunge (15 reps each leg)	Legs, Glutes, Core	Step forward, lower hips to drop knee to ground. Perform 15 reps each leg.
	(2) Pike Push-Up (10 reps)	Shoulders, Triceps, Core	Push-up with hips high, resembles downward dog pose. Perform 10 reps.
	(3) Russian Twist (20 reps)	Core, Obliques, Hip Flexors	Twist torso holding weight, seated on ground. Perform 20 reps.
36	**30 seconds work, 30 seconds rest per exercise for 4 rounds:**		
	(1) Mountain Climbers	Core, Legs, Shoulders	Run in place in plank position, drive knees to chest. Perform for 45 seconds.
	(2) Side Crunches	Core, Obliques, Hip Flexors	Lie on side, perform crunches towards elevated leg. Perform for 45 seconds.
	(3) Jumping Jacks	Full Body, Cardio, Legs	Jump to spread legs and clap hands overhead. Perform for 45 seconds.
	(4) Walking Lunges	Legs, Glutes, Core	Step forward into a lunge, move forward alternating legs. Perform for 45 seconds.
37	**As many rounds as possible in 10 mins of:**		
	(1) Burpees (10 reps)	Full Body, Core, Legs	Jump, squat down, kick back into a push-up, return up. Perform 10 reps.
	(2) Plank Rotation (10 reps each side)	Core, Shoulders, Obliques	Rotate body in plank, extend arm upward, switch sides. Perform 10 reps each side.
	(3) Calf Raises (20 reps)	Calves, Core, Balance	Lift heels off ground, balance on toes, lower slowly. Perform 20 reps.
38	**As many rounds as possible in 12 mins:**		
	(1) High Knees (30 seconds)	Legs, Core, Cardio	Run in place lifting knees high, maintain pace. Perform for 30 seconds.
	(2) Scissor Kicks (30 seconds)	Core, Hip Flexors, Lower Abs	Alternately lift legs in lying position, engages core. Perform for 30 seconds.
	(3) Jumping Jacks (30 seconds)	Full Body, Cardio, Legs	Jump to spread legs and clap hands overhead. Perform for 30 seconds.

Workout No.	Workout	Main Muscle Groups	Instructions
39	**Every minute on the minute for 20 mins:**		
	(1) Pull-Ups (5 reps)	Back, Biceps, Shoulders	Pull body up on bar, chin above hands. Perform 5 reps.
	(2) Hip Raise (10 reps)	Glutes, Core, Hamstrings	Lift hips while lying on back, feet flat on ground. Perform 10 reps.
	(3) Fire Hydrants (10 reps each leg)	Glutes, Core, Hip Flexors	On hands and knees, lift leg to side, keep knee bent. Perform 10 reps each leg.
40	**45 seconds work, 15 seconds rest per exercise for 4 rounds:**		
	(1) High Knees	Legs, Core, Cardio	Run in place lifting knees high, maintain pace. Perform for 45 seconds.
	(2) Bear Crawl	Full Body, Core, Shoulders	Crawl forward on all fours, hips down, move quickly. Perform for 45 seconds.
	(3) Flutter Kicks	Core, Hip Flexors, Lower Abs	Lie on back, alternately kick legs in small, rapid motion. Perform for 45 seconds.
	(4) Crab Walk	Triceps, Core, Glutes	Walk backward on hands and feet, hips elevated. Perform for 45 seconds.
41	**As many rounds as possible in 10 mins of:**		
	(1) Alternate Arm/Leg Plank (10 reps each side)	Core, Shoulders, Glutes	Plank, extend opposite arm and leg, hold. Perform 10 reps each side.
	(2) Bodyweight Row (15 reps)	Back, Biceps, Core	Pull body up towards a bar or table, lying underneath. Perform 15 reps.
	(3) Walking Toe Touches (20 meters)	Hamstrings, Core, Shoulders	Walk, reach down to touch toes with opposite hand. Perform 20 meters.
42	**45 seconds work, 15 seconds rest per exercise for 4 rounds:**		
	(1) High Knees	Legs, Core, Cardio	Run in place lifting knees high, maintain pace. Perform for 45 seconds.
	(2) Cross-Body Crunches	Core, Obliques, Hip Flexors	Touch opposite knee to elbow, lying down. Perform for 45 seconds.
	(3) Jumping Jacks	Full Body, Cardio, Legs	Jump to spread legs and clap hands overhead. Perform for 45 seconds.
	(4) Bird Dog	Core, Glutes, Shoulders	Extend opposite arm and leg, kneeling position. Perform for 45 seconds.
43	**Every minute on the minute for 20 mins:**		
	(1) Push-Ups (10 reps)	Chest, Triceps, Shoulders	Lower body to ground, push up with arms. Perform 10 reps.
	(2) Glute Bridge (15 reps)	Glutes, Core, Hamstrings	Lift hips while lying on back, feet flat on ground. Perform 15 reps.
	(3) Side Plank (30 seconds each side)	Core, Shoulders, Obliques	Support body on one arm, side facing ground. Hold for 30 seconds each side.
44	**As many rounds as possible in 12 mins:**		
	(1) Tuck Jumps (10 reps)	Legs, Core, Cardio	Jump high, tuck knees to chest mid-air. Perform 10 reps.
	(2) Fire Hydrant (15 reps each leg)	Glutes, Core, Hip Flexors	On hands and knees, lift leg to side, keep knee bent. Perform 15 reps each leg.
	(3) Plank Rotation (10 reps each side)	Core, Shoulders, Obliques	Rotate body in plank, extend arm upward, switch sides. Perform 10 reps each side.

Workout No.	Workout	Main Muscle Groups	Instructions
45	**5 Rounds for time:**		
	(1) Inchworm (10 reps)	Full Body, Core, Shoulders	Walk hands forward from standing, hold plank, walk back. Perform 10 reps.
	(2) Single Leg Split Squat (10 reps each leg)	Quads, Glutes, Core	Perform split squat on one leg, elevated rear foot. Perform 10 reps each leg.
	(3) Dolphin Kick (15 reps)	Core, Glutes, Hamstrings	Lie face down, kick legs like a dolphin's tail. Perform 15 reps.
46	**40 seconds work, 20 seconds rest per exercise for 4 rounds:**		
	(1) Mountain Climbers	Core, Legs, Shoulders	Run in place in plank position, drive knees to chest. Perform for 45 seconds.
	(2) Side Crunches	Core, Obliques, Hip Flexors	Lie on side, perform crunches towards elevated leg. Perform for 45 seconds.
	(3) Calf Raises	Calves, Core, Balance	Lift heels off ground, balance on toes, lower slowly. Perform for 45 seconds.
	(4) Crab Toe Touch	Core, Triceps, Glutes	Crab walk position, touch opposite foot with hand. Perform for 45 seconds.
47	**As many rounds as possible in 10 mins of:**		
	(1) Burpees (10 reps)	Full Body, Core, Legs	Jump, squat down, kick back into a push-up, return up. Perform 10 reps.
	(2) Side-to-Side Push-Up (10 reps each side)	Chest, Shoulders, Core	Shift side-to-side during push-ups, engages core. Perform 10 reps each side.
	(3) Windshield Wipers (15 reps)	Core, Obliques, Hip Flexors	Swing legs side-to-side lying down, mimic wiper. Perform 15 reps.
48	**As many rounds as possible in 12 mins:**		
	(1) High Knees (30 seconds)	Legs, Core, Cardio	Run in place lifting knees high, maintain pace. Perform for 30 seconds.
	(2) Bear Crawl (30 seconds)	Full Body, Core, Shoulders	Crawl forward on all fours, hips down, move quickly. Perform for 30 seconds.
	(3) Jumping Jacks (30 seconds)	Full Body, Cardio, Legs	Jump to spread legs and clap hands overhead. Perform for 30 seconds.
49	**Every minute on the minute for 20 mins:**		
	(1) Pull-Ups (5 reps)	Back, Biceps, Shoulders	Pull body up on bar, chin above hands. Perform 5 reps.
	(2) Hip Raise (10 reps)	Glutes, Core, Hamstrings	Lift hips while lying on back, feet flat on ground. Perform 10 reps.
	(3) Spiderman (10 reps each side)	Core, Shoulders, Legs	Bring knee to elbow during push-up, switch sides. Perform 10 reps each side.
50	**45 seconds work, 15 seconds rest per exercise for 4 rounds:**		
	(1) High Knees	Legs, Core, Cardio	Run in place lifting knees high, maintain pace. Perform for 45 seconds.
	(2) Bodyweight Row	Back, Biceps, Core	Pull body up towards a bar or table, lying underneath. Perform for 45 seconds.
	(3) Flutter Kicks	Core, Hip Flexors, Lower Abs	Lie on back, alternately kick legs in small, rapid motion. Perform for 45 seconds.
	(4) Side Lunge	Legs, Glutes, Core	Step to side into lunge, keep other leg straight. Perform for 45 seconds.

Workout No.	Workout	Main Muscle Groups	Instructions
51	**As many rounds as possible in 10 mins of:**		
	(1) Burpees (15 reps)	Full Body, Core, Legs	Jump, squat down, kick back into a push-up, return up. Perform 15 reps.
	(2) Hanging Knee Raise (10 reps)	Core, Hip Flexors, Back	Hang from bar, raise knees towards chest. Perform 10 reps.
	(3) Side Lunges (12 reps each side)	Legs, Glutes, Core	Step to side into lunge, keep other leg straight. Perform 12 reps each side.
52	**50 seconds work, 10 seconds rest per exercise for 4 rounds:**		
	(1) High Knees	Legs, Core, Cardio	Run in place lifting knees high, maintain pace. Perform for 45 seconds.
	(2) Cross-Body Crunches	Core, Obliques, Hip Flexors	Touch opposite knee to elbow, lying down. Perform for 45 seconds.
	(3) Jumping Jacks	Full Body, Cardio, Legs	Jump to spread legs and clap hands overhead. Perform for 45 seconds.
	(4) Tricep Dips	Triceps, Shoulders, Core	Dip body between bars, focus on triceps. Perform for 45 seconds.
53	**Every minute on the minute for 20 mins:**		
	(1) Pike Push-Ups (10 reps)	Shoulders, Triceps, Core	Push-up with hips high, resembles downward dog pose. Perform 10 reps.
	(2) Lying Leg Lift (15 reps)	Core, Lower Abs, Hip Flexors	Raise legs vertically, lying flat on back. Perform 15 reps.
	(3) Crab Walk (20 meters)	Triceps, Core, Glutes	Walk backward on hands and feet, hips elevated. Perform 20 meters.
54	**As many rounds as possible in 12 mins:**		
	(1) Tuck Jumps (10 reps)	Legs, Core, Cardio	Jump high, tuck knees to chest mid-air. Perform 10 reps.
	(2) Fire Hydrant (15 reps each leg)	Glutes, Core, Hip Flexors	On hands and knees, lift leg to side, keep knee bent. Perform 15 reps each leg.
	(3) Plank Rotation (10 reps each side)	Core, Shoulders, Obliques	Rotate body in plank, extend arm upward, switch sides. Perform 10 reps each side.
55	**5 Rounds for time:**		
	(1) Inchworm (10 reps)	Full Body, Core, Shoulders	Walk hands forward from standing, hold plank, walk back. Perform 10 reps.
	(2) Single Leg Dead Lift (10 reps each leg)	Hamstrings, Glutes, Core	Balance on one leg, hinge forward, extend free leg back. Perform 10 reps each leg.
	(3) Reverse Crunch (15 reps)	Core, Hip Flexors, Lower Abs	Lift hips off floor, knees towards chest. Perform 15 reps.
56	**45 seconds work, 15 seconds rest per exercise for 4 rounds:**		
	(1) Mountain Climbers	Core, Legs, Shoulders	Run in place in plank position, drive knees to chest. Perform for 45 seconds.
	(2) Side Crunches	Core, Obliques, Hip Flexors	Lie on side, perform crunches towards elevated leg. Perform for 45 seconds.
	(3) Calf Raises	Calves, Core, Balance	Lift heels off ground, balance on toes, lower slowly. Perform for 45 seconds.
	(4) Skater Squat	Legs, Glutes, Core	Balance on one leg, squat, touch opposite hand to foot. Perform for 45 seconds.

Workout No.	Workout		Main Muscle Groups	Instructions
57	As many rounds as possible in 10 mins of:			
	(1)	Box Jumps (15 reps)	Legs, Glutes, Core	Jump onto and off a box repeatedly, land softly. Perform 15 reps.
	(2)	Side Plank (30 seconds each side)	Core, Shoulders, Obliques	Support body on one arm, side facing ground. Hold for 30 seconds each side.
	(3)	Bird Dog (10 reps each side)	Core, Glutes, Shoulders	Extend opposite arm and leg, kneeling position. Perform 10 reps each side.
58	As many rounds as possible in 12 mins:			
	(1)	High Knees (30 seconds)	Legs, Core, Cardio	Run in place lifting knees high, maintain pace. Perform for 30 seconds.
	(2)	Dolphin Kick (30 seconds)	Core, Glutes, Hamstrings	Lie face down, kick legs like a dolphin's tail. Perform for 30 seconds.
	(3)	Jumping Jacks (30 seconds)	Full Body, Cardio, Legs	Jump to spread legs and clap hands overhead. Perform for 30 seconds.
59	Every minute on the minute for 20 mins:			
	(1)	Pull-Ups (5 reps)	Back, Biceps, Shoulders	Pull body up on bar, chin above hands. Perform 5 reps.
	(2)	Hip Raise (10 reps)	Glutes, Core, Hamstrings	Lift hips while lying on back, feet flat on ground. Perform 10 reps.
	(3)	Spiderman (10 reps each side)	Core, Shoulders, Legs	Bring knee to elbow during push-up, switch sides. Perform 10 reps each side.
60	45 seconds work, 15 seconds rest per exercise for 4 rounds:			
	(1)	High Knees	Legs, Core, Cardio	Run in place lifting knees high, maintain pace. Perform for 45 seconds.
	(2)	Bodyweight Row	Back, Biceps, Core	Pull body up towards a bar or table, lying underneath. Perform for 45 seconds.
	(3)	Flutter Kicks	Core, Hip Flexors, Lower Abs	Lie on back, alternately kick legs in small, rapid motion. Perform for 45 seconds.
	(4)	Side Lunge	Legs, Glutes, Core	Step to side into lunge, keep other leg straight. Perform for 45 seconds.
61	As many rounds as possible in 10 mins of:			
	(1)	Fire Hydrant (15 reps each leg)	Glutes, Core, Hip Flexors	On hands and knees, lift leg to side, keep knee bent. Perform 15 reps each leg.
	(2)	Superman (15 reps)	Lower Back, Glutes, Shoulders	Extend arms and legs while face down, hold position. Perform 15 reps.
	(3)	Burpees (10 reps)	Full Body, Core, Legs	Jump, squat down, kick back into a push-up, return up. Perform 10 reps.
62	30 seconds work, 30 seconds rest per exercise for 4 rounds:			
	(1)	High Knees	Legs, Core, Cardio	Run in place lifting knees high, maintain pace. Perform for 45 seconds.
	(2)	Cross-Body Crunches	Core, Obliques, Hip Flexors	Touch opposite knee to elbow, lying down. Perform for 45 seconds.
	(3)	Jumping Jacks	Full Body, Cardio, Legs	Jump to spread legs and clap hands overhead. Perform for 45 seconds.
	(4)	Bodyweight Row	Back, Biceps, Core	Pull body up towards a bar or table, lying underneath. Perform for 45 seconds.

Workout No.	Workout	Main Muscle Groups	Instructions
63	**Every minute on the minute for 20 mins:**		
	(1) Push-Ups (10 reps)	Chest, Triceps, Shoulders	Lower body to ground, push up with arms. Perform 10 reps.
	(2) Side Plank (30 seconds each side)	Core, Shoulders, Obliques	Support body on one arm, side facing ground. Hold for 30 seconds each side.
	(3) Flutter Kicks (15 reps)	Core, Hip Flexors, Lower Abs	Lie on back, alternately kick legs in small, rapid motion. Perform 15 reps.
64	**As many rounds as possible in 12 mins:**		
	(1) Tuck Jumps (10 reps)	Legs, Core, Cardio	Jump high, tuck knees to chest mid-air. Perform 10 reps.
	(2) Bird Dog (10 reps each side)	Core, Glutes, Shoulders	Extend opposite arm and leg, kneeling position. Perform 10 reps each side.
	(3) Plank (30 seconds)	Core, Shoulders, Back	Hold body straight on elbows, maintain line. Perform for 30 seconds.
65	**5 Rounds for time:**		
	(1) Inchworm (10 reps)	Full Body, Core, Shoulders	Walk hands forward from standing, hold plank, walk back. Perform 10 reps.
	(2) Single Leg Squat (10 reps each leg)	Quads, Glutes, Core	Stand on one leg, squat, maintain balance. Perform 10 reps each leg.
	(3) Dolphin Kick (15 reps)	Core, Glutes, Hamstrings	Lie face down, kick legs like a dolphin's tail. Perform 15 reps.
66	**45 seconds work, 15 seconds rest per exercise for 4 rounds:**		
	(1) Mountain Climbers	Core, Legs, Shoulders	Run in place in plank position, drive knees to chest. Perform for 45 seconds.
	(2) Side Crunches	Core, Obliques, Hip Flexors	Lie on side, perform crunches towards elevated leg. Perform for 45 seconds.
	(3) Calf Raises	Calves, Core, Balance	Lift heels off ground, balance on toes, lower slowly. Perform for 45 seconds.
	(4) Crab Toe Touch	Core, Triceps, Glutes	Crab walk position, touch opposite foot with hand. Perform for 45 seconds.
67	**As many rounds as possible in 10 mins of:**		
	(1) Bear Crawl (20 meters)	Full Body, Core, Shoulders	Crawl forward on all fours, hips down, move quickly. Perform 20 meters.
	(2) Side-to-Side Push-Up (10 reps each side)	Chest, Shoulders, Core	Shift side-to-side during push-ups, engages core. Perform 10 reps each side.
	(3) Windshield Wipers (15 reps)	Core, Obliques, Hip Flexors	Swing legs side-to-side lying down, mimic wiper. Perform 15 reps.
68	**As many rounds as possible in 12 mins:**		
	(1) High Knees (30 seconds)	Legs, Core, Cardio	Run in place lifting knees high, maintain pace. Perform for 30 seconds.
	(2) Bear Crawl (30 seconds)	Full Body, Core, Shoulders	Crawl forward on all fours, hips down, move quickly. Perform for 30 seconds.
	(3) Jumping Jacks (30 seconds)	Full Body, Cardio, Legs	Jump to spread legs and clap hands overhead. Perform for 30 seconds.

Workout No.	Workout	Main Muscle Groups	Instructions
69	**Every minute on the minute for 20 mins:**		
	(1) Pull-Ups (5 reps)	Back, Biceps, Shoulders	Pull body up on bar, chin above hands. Perform 5 reps.
	(2) Hip Raise (10 reps)	Glutes, Core, Hamstrings	Lift hips while lying on back, feet flat on ground. Perform 10 reps.
	(3) Spiderman (10 reps each side)	Core, Shoulders, Legs	Bring knee to elbow during push-up, switch sides. Perform 10 reps each side.
70	**45 seconds work, 15 seconds rest per exercise for 4 rounds:**		
	(1) High Knees	Legs, Core, Cardio	Run in place lifting knees high, maintain pace. Perform for 45 seconds.
	(2) Cross-Body Crunch	Core, Obliques, Hip Flexors	Touch opposite knee to elbow, lying down. Perform for 45 seconds.
	(3) Jumping Jacks	Full Body, Cardio, Legs	Jump to spread legs and clap hands overhead. Perform for 45 seconds.
	(4) Skater Squat	Legs, Glutes, Core	Balance on one leg, squat, touch opposite hand to foot. Perform for 45 seconds.
71	**As many rounds as possible in 10 mins of:**		
	(1) Lunge (15 reps each leg)	Legs, Glutes, Core	Step forward, lower hips to drop knee to ground. Perform 15 reps each leg.
	(2) Plank Rotation (10 reps each side)	Core, Shoulders, Obliques	Rotate body in plank, extend arm upward, switch sides. Perform 10 reps each side.
	(3) Glute Bridge (20 reps)	Glutes, Core, Hamstrings	Lift hips while lying on back, feet flat on ground. Perform 20 reps.
72	**40 seconds work, 20 seconds rest per exercise for 4 rounds:**		
	(1) High Knees	Legs, Core, Cardio	Run in place lifting knees high, maintain pace. Perform for 45 seconds.
	(2) Bear Crawl	Full Body, Core, Shoulders	Crawl forward on all fours, hips down, move quickly. Perform for 45 seconds.
	(3) Flutter Kicks	Core, Hip Flexors, Lower Abs	Lie on back, alternately kick legs in small, rapid motion. Perform for 45 seconds.
	(4) Side Plank	Core, Shoulders, Obliques	Support body on one arm, side facing ground. Perform for 45 seconds each side.
73	**Every minute on the minute for 20 mins:**		
	(1) Pike Push-Ups (10 reps)	Shoulders, Triceps, Core	Push-up with hips high, resembles downward dog pose. Perform 10 reps.
	(2) Side Lunges (15 reps each leg)	Legs, Glutes, Core	Step to side into lunge, keep other leg straight. Perform 15 reps each leg.
	(3) Mountain Climbers (20 reps)	Core, Legs, Shoulders	Run in place in plank position, drive knees to chest. Perform 20 reps.
74	**As many rounds as possible in 12 mins:**		
	(1) Tuck Jumps (10 reps)	Legs, Core, Cardio	Jump high, tuck knees to chest mid-air. Perform 10 reps.
	(2) Bird Dog (10 reps each side)	Core, Glutes, Shoulders	Extend opposite arm and leg, kneeling position. Perform 10 reps each side.
	(3) Plank (30 seconds)	Core, Shoulders, Back	Hold body straight on elbows, maintain line. Perform for 30 seconds.

Workout No.	Workout	Main Muscle Groups	Instructions
75	**5 Rounds for time:**		
	(1) Inchworm (10 reps)	Full Body, Core, Shoulders	Walk hands forward from standing, hold plank, walk back. Perform 10 reps.
	(2) Single Leg Dead Lift (10 reps each leg)	Hamstrings, Glutes, Core	Balance on one leg, hinge forward, extend free leg back. Perform 10 reps each leg.
	(3) Cross-Body Crunch (20 reps)	Core, Obliques, Hip Flexors	Touch opposite knee to elbow, lying down. Perform 20 reps.
	(4) Bodyweight Row (3 rounds of 10 reps)	Back, Biceps, Core	Pull body up towards a bar, lying underneath. Keep a straight body line.
	(5) Bicycle Crunches (3 rounds of 20 reps)	Abs, Obliques, Hip Flexors	Alternate elbows to opposite knees. Keep the motion controlled and steady.
76	**45 seconds work, 15 seconds rest per exercise for 4 rounds:**		
	(1) Mountain Climbers	Core, Legs, Shoulders	Run in place in plank position, drive knees to chest. Perform for 45 seconds.
	(2) Side Crunches	Core, Obliques, Hip Flexors	Lie on side, perform crunches towards elevated leg. Perform for 45 seconds.
	(3) Calf Raises	Calves, Core, Balance	Lift heels off ground, balance on toes, lower slowly. Perform for 45 seconds.
	(4) Crab Walk	Triceps, Core, Glutes	Walk backward on hands and feet, hips elevated. Perform for 45 seconds.
77	**As many rounds as possible in 10 mins of:**		
	(1) Burpees (10 reps)	Full Body, Core, Legs	Jump, squat down, kick back into a push-up, return up. Perform 10 reps.
	(2) Side-to-Side Push-Up (10 reps each side)	Chest, Shoulders, Core	Shift side-to-side during push-ups, engages core. Perform 10 reps each side.
	(3) Windshield Wipers (15 reps)	Core, Obliques, Hip Flexors	Swing legs side-to-side lying down, mimic wiper. Perform 15 reps.
78	**As many rounds as possible in 12 mins:**		
	(1) High Knees (30 seconds)	Legs, Core, Cardio	Run in place lifting knees high, maintain pace. Perform for 30 seconds.
	(2) Dolphin Kick (30 seconds)	Core, Glutes, Hamstrings	Lie face down, kick legs like a dolphin's tail. Perform for 30 seconds.
	(3) Jumping Jacks (30 seconds)	Full Body, Cardio, Legs	Jump to spread legs and clap hands overhead. Perform for 30 seconds.
79	**Every minute on the minute for 20 mins:**		
	(1) Pull-Ups (5 reps)	Back, Biceps, Shoulders	Pull body up on bar, chin above hands. Perform 5 reps.
	(2) Hip Raise (10 reps)	Glutes, Core, Hamstrings	Lift hips while lying on back, feet flat on ground. Perform 10 reps.
	(3) Spiderman (10 reps each side)	Core, Shoulders, Legs	Bring knee to elbow during push-up, switch sides. Perform 10 reps each side.
80	**50 seconds work, 10 seconds rest per exercise for 4 rounds:**		
	(1) High Knees	Legs, Core, Cardio	Run in place lifting knees high, maintain pace. Perform for 45 seconds.
	(2) Cross-Body Crunch	Core, Obliques, Hip Flexors	Touch opposite knee to elbow, lying down. Perform for 45 seconds.
	(3) Jumping Jacks	Full Body, Cardio, Legs	Jump to spread legs and clap hands overhead. Perform for 45 seconds.
	(4) Skater Squat	Legs, Glutes, Core	Balance on one leg, squat, touch opposite hand to foot. Perform for 45 seconds.

Workout No.	Workout	Main Muscle Groups	Instructions
81	**As many rounds as possible in 10 mins of:**		
	(1) Plank to Push-Up (10 reps)	Core, Shoulders, Triceps	Alternate between plank and push-up positions. Perform 10 reps.
	(2) Step-Ups (15 reps each leg)	Legs, Glutes, Core	Step onto a raised platform, alternate legs. Perform 15 reps each leg.
	(3) Bicycle Crunches (20 reps)	Core, Obliques, Hip Flexors	Lie down, alternate elbows to opposite knees cycling legs. Perform 20 reps.
82	**45 seconds work, 15 seconds rest per exercise for 4 rounds:**		
	(1) High Knees	Legs, Core, Cardio	Run in place lifting knees high, maintain pace. Perform for 45 seconds.
	(2) Plank Jacks	Core, Shoulders, Cardio	Jump feet in and out while holding a plank position. Perform for 45 seconds.
	(3) Squat Jumps	Legs, Glutes, Cardio	Perform a squat then jump explosively. Perform for 45 seconds.
	(4) Russian Twists	Core, Obliques, Hip Flexors	Twist torso holding weight, seated on ground. Perform for 45 seconds.
83	**Every minute on the minute for 20 mins:**		
	(1) Pull-Ups (5 reps)	Back, Biceps, Shoulders	Pull body up on bar, chin above hands. Perform 5 reps.
	(2) Side Plank with Leg Lift (10 reps each side)	Core, Glutes, Shoulders	Hold side plank, lift top leg, lower slowly. Perform 10 reps each side.
	(3) Donkey Kicks (15 reps each leg)	Glutes, Core, Hamstrings	On hands and knees, kick one leg back and up. Perform 15 reps each leg.
84	**As many rounds as possible in 12 mins:**		
	(1) Tuck Jumps (10 reps)	Legs, Core, Cardio	Jump high, tuck knees to chest mid-air. Perform 10 reps.
	(2) Bird Dog (10 reps each side)	Core, Glutes, Shoulders	Extend opposite arm and leg, kneeling position. Perform 10 reps each side.
	(3) Plank (30 seconds)	Core, Shoulders, Back	Hold body straight on elbows, maintain line. Perform for 30 seconds.
85	**5 Rounds for time:**		
	(1) Burpees (10 reps)	Full Body, Core, Legs	Jump, squat down, kick back into a push-up, return up. Perform 10 reps.
	(2) Single Leg Squat (10 reps each leg)	Quads, Glutes, Core	Stand on one leg, squat, maintain balance. Perform 10 reps each leg.
	(3) Cross-Body Mountain Climbers (15 reps each side)	Core, Shoulders, Cardio	Bring knee towards opposite elbow while in plank position. Perform 15 reps each side.
86	**50 seconds work, 10 seconds rest per exercise for 4 rounds:**		
	(1) Jumping Jacks	Full Body, Cardio, Legs	Jump to spread legs and clap hands overhead. Perform for 45 seconds.
	(2) Plank with Shoulder Tap	Core, Shoulders, Triceps	In plank position, tap opposite shoulder with each hand. Perform for 45 seconds.
	(3) Glute Bridge March	Glutes, Core, Hamstrings	Lift hips into bridge, alternate lifting each knee towards chest. Perform for 45 seconds.
	(4) Flutter Kicks	Core, Hip Flexors, Lower Abs	Lie on back, alternately kick legs in small, rapid motion. Perform for 45 seconds.

Workout No.	Workout		Main Muscle Groups	Instructions
87	**As many rounds as possible in 10 mins of:**			
	(1)	Squat (20 reps)	Legs, Glutes, Core	Stand, bend knees to lower body, keep back straight. Perform 20 reps.
	(2)	Plank Rotation (10 reps each side)	Core, Shoulders, Obliques	Rotate body in plank, extend arm upward, switch sides. Perform 10 reps each side.
	(3)	Step-Ups (15 reps each leg)	Legs, Glutes, Core	Step onto a raised platform, alternate legs. Perform 15 reps each leg.
88	**As many rounds as possible in 12 mins:**			
	(1)	High Knees (30 seconds)	Legs, Core, Cardio	Run in place lifting knees high, maintain pace. Perform for 30 seconds.
	(2)	Bear Crawl (30 seconds)	Full Body, Core, Shoulders	Crawl forward on all fours, hips down, move quickly. Perform for 30 seconds.
	(3)	Jumping Jacks (30 seconds)	Full Body, Cardio, Legs	Jump to spread legs and clap hands overhead. Perform for 30 seconds.
89	**Every minute on the minute for 20 mins:**			
	(1)	Pull-Ups (5 reps)	Back, Biceps, Shoulders	Pull body up on bar, chin above hands. Perform 5 reps.
	(2)	Hip Raise (10 reps)	Glutes, Core, Hamstrings	Lift hips while lying on back, feet flat on ground. Perform 10 reps.
	(3)	Fire Hydrant (10 reps each leg)	Glutes, Core, Hip Flexors	On hands and knees, lift leg to side, keep knee bent. Perform 10 reps each leg.
90	**45 seconds work, 15 seconds rest per exercise for 4 rounds:**			
	(1)	High Knees	Legs, Core, Cardio	Run in place lifting knees high, maintain pace. Perform for 45 seconds.
	(2)	Cross-Body Crunch	Core, Obliques, Hip Flexors	Touch opposite knee to elbow, lying down. Perform for 45 seconds.
	(3)	Jumping Jacks	Full Body, Cardio, Legs	Jump to spread legs and clap hands overhead. Perform for 45 seconds.
	(4)	Skater Squat	Legs, Glutes, Core	Balance on one leg, squat, touch opposite hand to foot. Perform for 45 seconds.
91	**As many rounds as possible in 10 mins of:**			
	(1)	Alternating Lunges (15 reps each leg)	Legs, Glutes, Core	Step forward, lower hips to drop knee to ground. Perform 15 reps each leg.
	(2)	Push-Up with Extension (10 reps each side)	Chest, Shoulders, Core	Perform push up, extend one arm forward, alternate. Perform 10 reps each side.
	(3)	Flutter Kicks (20 reps)	Core, Hip Flexors, Lower Abs	Lie on back, alternately kick legs in small, rapid motion. Perform 20 reps.
92	**30 seconds work, 30 seconds rest per exercise for 4 rounds:**			
	(1)	High Knees	Legs, Core, Cardio	Run in place lifting knees high, maintain pace. Perform for 45 seconds.
	(2)	Burpees	Full Body, Core, Legs	Jump, squat down, kick back into a push-up, return up. Perform for 45 seconds.
	(3)	Plank to Push-Up	Core, Shoulders, Triceps	Alternate between plank and push-up positions. Perform for 45 seconds.
	(4)	Russian Twists	Core, Obliques, Hip Flexors	Twist torso holding weight, seated on ground. Perform for 45 seconds.

Workout No.	Workout	Main Muscle Groups	Instructions
93	Every minute on the minute for 20 mins:		
	(1) Pull-Ups (5 reps)	Back, Biceps, Shoulders	Pull body up on bar, chin above hands. Perform 5 reps.
	(2) Glute Bridge (15 reps)	Glutes, Core, Hamstrings	Lift hips while lying on back, feet flat on ground. Perform 15 reps.
	(3) Fire Hydrant (10 reps each leg)	Glutes, Core, Hip Flexors	On hands and knees, lift leg to side, keep knee bent. Perform 10 reps each leg.
94	As many rounds as possible in 12 mins:		
	(1) Tuck Jumps (10 reps)	Legs, Core, Cardio	Jump high, tuck knees to chest mid-air. Perform 10 reps.
	(2) Bird Dog (10 reps each side)	Core, Glutes, Shoulders	Extend opposite arm and leg, kneeling position. Perform 10 reps each side.
	(3) Plank Rotation (10 reps each side)	Core, Shoulders, Obliques	Rotate body in plank, extend arm upward, switch sides. Perform 10 reps each side.
95	5 Rounds for time:		
	(1) Inchworm (10 reps)	Full Body, Core, Shoulders	Walk hands forward from standing, hold plank, walk back. Perform 10 reps.
	(2) Single Leg Dead Lift (10 reps each leg)	Hamstrings, Glutes, Core	Balance on one leg, hinge forward, extend free leg back. Perform 10 reps each leg.
	(3) Reverse Crunch (15 reps)	Core, Hip Flexors, Lower Abs	Lift hips off floor, knees towards chest. Perform 15 reps.
96	45 seconds work, 15 seconds rest per exercise for 4 rounds:		
	(1) Mountain Climbers	Core, Legs, Shoulders	Run in place in plank position, drive knees to chest. Perform for 45 seconds.
	(2) Side Crunches	Core, Obliques, Hip Flexors	Lie on side, perform crunches towards elevated leg. Perform for 45 seconds.
	(3) Jumping Jacks	Full Body, Cardio, Legs	Jump to spread legs and clap hands overhead. Perform for 45 seconds.
	(4) Crab Walk	Triceps, Core, Glutes	Walk backward on hands and feet, hips elevated. Perform for 45 seconds.
97	As many rounds as possible in 10 mins of:		
	(1) Burpees (10 reps)	Full Body, Core, Legs	Jump, squat down, kick back into a push-up, return up. Perform 10 reps.
	(2) Side-to-Side Push-Up (10 reps each side)	Chest, Shoulders, Core	Shift side-to-side during push-ups, engages core. Perform 10 reps each side.
	(3) Windshield Wipers (15 reps)	Core, Obliques, Hip Flexors	Swing legs side-to-side lying down, mimic wiper. Perform 15 reps.
98	As many rounds as possible in 12 mins:		
	(1) High Knees (30 seconds)	Legs, Core, Cardio	Run in place lifting knees high, maintain pace. Perform for 30 seconds.
	(2) Bear Crawl (30 seconds)	Full Body, Core, Shoulders	Crawl forward on all fours, hips down, move quickly. Perform for 30 seconds.
	(3) Jumping Jacks (30 seconds)	Full Body, Cardio, Legs	Jump to spread legs and clap hands overhead. Perform for 30 seconds.

Workout No.	Workout		Main Muscle Groups	Instructions
99	**Every minute on the minute for 20 mins:**			
	(1)	Pull-Ups (5 reps)	Back, Biceps, Shoulders	Pull body up on bar, chin above hands. Perform 5 reps.
	(2)	Hip Raise (10 reps)	Glutes, Core, Hamstrings	Lift hips while lying on back, feet flat on ground. Perform 10 reps.
	(3)	Spiderman (10 reps each side)	Core, Shoulders, Legs	Bring knee to elbow during push-up, switch sides. Perform 10 reps each side.
100	**45 seconds work, 15 seconds rest per exercise for 4 rounds:**			
	(1)	High Knees	Legs, Core, Cardio	Run in place lifting knees high, maintain pace. Perform for 45 seconds.
	(2)	Cross-Body Crunch	Core, Obliques, Hip Flexors	Touch opposite knee to elbow, lying down. Perform for 45 seconds.
	(3)	Jumping Jacks	Full Body, Cardio, Legs	Jump to spread legs and clap hands overhead. Perform for 45 seconds.
	(4)	Skater Squat	Legs, Glutes, Core	Balance on one leg, squat, touch opposite hand to foot. Perform for 45 seconds.
101	**As many rounds as possible in 10 mins of:**			
	(1)	Plank to Push-Up (10 reps)	Core, Shoulders, Triceps	Alternate between plank and push-up positions. Perform 10 reps.
	(2)	Jumping Jacks (20 reps)	Full Body, Cardio, Legs	Jump to spread legs and clap hands overhead. Perform 20 reps.
	(3)	Walking Lunges (15 reps each leg)	Legs, Glutes, Core	Step forward into a lunge, move forward alternating legs. Perform 15 reps each leg.
102	**50 seconds work, 10 seconds rest per exercise for 5 rounds:**			
	(1)	High Knees	Legs, Core, Cardio	Run in place lifting knees high, maintain pace. Perform for 45 seconds.
	(2)	Crab Toe Touch	Core, Triceps, Glutes	Crab walk position, touch opposite foot with hand. Perform for 45 seconds.
	(3)	Mountain Climbers	Core, Legs, Shoulders	Run in place in plank position, drive knees to chest. Perform for 45 seconds.
	(4)	Bicycle Crunches	Core, Obliques, Hip Flexors	Lie down, alternate elbows to opposite knees cycling legs. Perform for 45 seconds.
103	**Every minute on the minute for 20 mins:**			
	(1)	Pull-Ups (5 reps)	Back, Biceps, Shoulders	Pull body up on bar, chin above hands. Perform 5 reps.
	(2)	V-Ups (10 reps)	Core, Hip Flexors, Lower Abs	Lie back, lift legs and torso simultaneously, form 'V'. Perform 10 reps.
	(3)	Donkey Kicks (15 reps each leg)	Glutes, Core, Hamstrings	On hands and knees, kick one leg back and up. Perform 15 reps each leg.
104	**As many rounds as possible in 12 mins:**			
	(1)	Tuck Jumps (10 reps)	Legs, Core, Cardio	Jump high, tuck knees to chest mid-air. Perform 10 reps.
	(2)	Bird Dog (10 reps each side)	Core, Glutes, Shoulders	Extend opposite arm and leg, kneeling position. Perform 10 reps each side.
	(3)	Plank (30 seconds)	Core, Shoulders, Back	Hold body straight on elbows, maintain line. Perform for 30 seconds.

Workout No.		Workout	Main Muscle Groups	Instructions
105		**5 Rounds for time:**		
	(1)	Burpees (10 reps)	Full Body, Core, Legs	Jump, squat down, kick back into a push-up, return up. Perform 10 reps.
	(2)	Single Leg Squat (10 reps each leg)	Quads, Glutes, Core	Stand on one leg, squat, maintain balance. Perform 10 reps each leg.
	(3)	Cross-Body Mountain Climbers (15 reps each side)	Core, Shoulders, Cardio	Bring knee towards opposite elbow while in plank position. Perform 15 reps each side.
106		**30 seconds work, 30 seconds rest per exercise for 8 rounds:**		
	(1)	Jumping Jacks	Full Body, Cardio, Legs	Jump to spread legs and clap hands overhead. Perform for 45 seconds.
	(2)	Plank with Shoulder Tap	Core, Shoulders, Triceps	In plank position, tap opposite shoulder with each hand. Perform for 45 seconds.
	(3)	Glute Bridge March	Glutes, Core, Hamstrings	Lift hips into bridge, alternate lifting each knee towards chest. Perform for 45 seconds.
	(4)	Flutter Kicks	Core, Hip Flexors, Lower Abs	Lie on back, alternately kick legs in small, rapid motion. Perform for 45 seconds.
107		**As many rounds as possible in 10 mins of:**		
	(1)	Squat (20 reps)	Legs, Glutes, Core	Stand, bend knees to lower body, keep back straight. Perform 20 reps.
	(2)	Plank Rotation (10 reps each side)	Core, Shoulders, Obliques	Rotate body in plank, extend arm upward, switch sides. Perform 10 reps each side.
	(3)	Step-Ups (15 reps each leg)	Legs, Glutes, Core	Step onto a raised platform, alternate legs. Perform 15 reps each leg.
108		**As many rounds as possible in 12 mins:**		
	(1)	High Knees (30 seconds)	Legs, Core, Cardio	Run in place lifting knees high, maintain pace. Perform for 30 seconds.
	(2)	Bear Crawl (30 seconds)	Full Body, Core, Shoulders	Crawl forward on all fours, hips down, move quickly. Perform for 30 seconds.
	(3)	Jumping Jacks (30 seconds)	Full Body, Cardio, Legs	Jump to spread legs and clap hands overhead. Perform for 30 seconds.
109		**Every minute on the minute for 20 mins:**		
	(1)	Pull-Ups (5 reps)	Back, Biceps, Shoulders	Pull body up on bar, chin above hands. Perform 5 reps.
	(2)	Hip Raise (10 reps)	Glutes, Core, Hamstrings	Lift hips while lying on back, feet flat on ground. Perform 10 reps.
	(3)	Fire Hydrant (10 reps each leg)	Glutes, Core, Hip Flexors	On hands and knees, lift leg to side, keep knee bent. Perform 10 reps each leg.
110		**45 seconds work, 15 seconds rest per exercise for 5 rounds:**		
	(1)	High Knees	Legs, Core, Cardio	Run in place lifting knees high, maintain pace. Perform for 45 seconds.
	(2)	Cross-Body Crunch	Core, Obliques, Hip Flexors	Touch opposite knee to elbow, lying down. Perform for 45 seconds.
	(3)	Jumping Jacks	Full Body, Cardio, Legs	Jump to spread legs and clap hands overhead. Perform for 45 seconds.
	(4)	Skater Squat	Legs, Glutes, Core	Balance on one leg, squat, touch opposite hand to foot. Perform for 45 seconds.

Workout No.	Workout	Main Muscle Groups	Instructions
111	As many rounds as possible in 10 mins of:		
	(1) Box Jumps (15 reps)	Legs, Glutes, Core	Jump onto and off a box repeatedly, land softly. Perform 15 reps.
	(2) Pike Push-Ups (10 reps)	Shoulders, Triceps, Core	Push-up with hips high, resembles downward dog pose. Perform 10 reps.
	(3) Bicycle Crunches (20 reps)	Core, Obliques, Hip Flexors	Lie down, alternate elbows to opposite knees cycling legs. Perform 20 reps.
112	50 seconds work, 10 seconds rest per exercise for 5 rounds:		
	(1) High Knees	Legs, Core, Cardio	Run in place lifting knees high, maintain pace. Perform for 45 seconds.
	(2) Russian Twists	Core, Obliques, Hip Flexors	Twist torso holding weight, seated on ground. Perform for 45 seconds.
	(3) Burpees	Full Body, Core, Legs	Jump, squat down, kick back into a push-up, return up. Perform for 45 seconds.
	(4) Skater Squats	Legs, Glutes, Core	Balance on one leg, squat, touch opposite hand to foot. Perform for 45 seconds.
113	Every minute on the minute for 20 mins:		
	(1) Pull-Ups (5 reps)	Back, Biceps, Shoulders	Pull body up on bar, chin above hands. Perform 5 reps.
	(2) V-Ups (10 reps)	Core, Hip Flexors, Lower Abs	Lie back, lift legs and torso simultaneously, form 'V'. Perform 10 reps.
	(3) Side Lunges (10 reps each side)	Legs, Glutes, Core	Step to side into lunge, keep other leg straight. Perform 10 reps each side.
114	As many rounds as possible in 12 mins:		
	(1) Tuck Jumps (10 reps)	Legs, Core, Cardio	Jump high, tuck knees to chest mid-air. Perform 10 reps.
	(2) Plank with Shoulder Tap (10 reps each side)	Core, Shoulders, Triceps	In plank position, tap opposite shoulder with each hand. Perform 10 reps each side.
	(3) Jumping Jacks (20 reps)	Full Body, Cardio, Legs	Jump to spread legs and clap hands overhead. Perform 20 reps.
115	5 Rounds for time:		
	(1) Inchworm (10 reps)	Full Body, Core, Shoulders	Walk hands forward from standing, hold plank, walk back. Perform 10 reps.
	(2) Single Leg Dead Lift (10 reps each leg)	Hamstrings, Glutes, Core	Balance on one leg, hinge forward, extend free leg back. Perform 10 reps each leg.
	(3) Cross-Body Mountain Climbers (15 reps each side)	Core, Shoulders, Cardio	Bring knee towards opposite elbow while in plank position. Perform 15 reps each side.
116	30 seconds work, 30 seconds rest per exercise for 6 rounds:		
	(1) Jumping Jacks	Full Body, Cardio, Legs	Jump to spread legs and clap hands overhead. Perform for 45 seconds.
	(2) Crab Walk	Triceps, Core, Glutes	Walk backward on hands and feet, hips elevated. Perform for 45 seconds.
	(3) Flutter Kicks	Core, Hip Flexors, Lower Abs	Lie on back, alternately kick legs in small, rapid motion. Perform for 45 seconds.
	(4) Donkey Kicks	Glutes, Core, Hamstrings	On hands and knees, kick one leg back and up. Perform for 45 seconds.

Workout No.	Workout	Main Muscle Groups	Instructions
117	**As many rounds as possible in 10 mins of:**		
	(1) Burpees (10 reps)	Full Body, Core, Legs	Jump, squat down, kick back into a push-up, return up. Perform 10 reps.
	(2) Plank Rotation (10 reps each side)	Core, Shoulders, Obliques	Rotate body in plank, extend arm upward, switch sides. Perform 10 reps each side.
	(3) Step-Ups (15 reps each leg)	Legs, Glutes, Core	Step onto a raised platform, alternate legs. Perform 15 reps each leg.
118	**As many rounds as possible in 12 mins:**		
	(1) High Knees (30 seconds)	Legs, Core, Cardio	Run in place lifting knees high, maintain pace. Perform for 30 seconds.
	(2) Side-to-Side Push-Ups (10 reps each side)	Chest, Shoulders, Core	Shift side-to-side during push-ups, engages core. Perform 10 reps each side.
	(3) Jumping Jacks (30 seconds)	Full Body, Cardio, Legs	Jump to spread legs and clap hands overhead. Perform for 30 seconds.
119	**Every minute on the minute for 20 mins:**		
	(1) Pull-Ups (5 reps)	Back, Biceps, Shoulders	Pull body up on bar, chin above hands. Perform 5 reps.
	(2) Hip Raise (10 reps)	Glutes, Core, Hamstrings	Lift hips while lying on back, feet flat on ground. Perform 10 reps.
	(3) Fire Hydrant (10 reps each leg)	Glutes, Core, Hip Flexors	On hands and knees, lift leg to side, keep knee bent. Perform 10 reps each leg.
120	**45 seconds work, 15 seconds rest per exercise for 5 rounds:**		
	(1) High Knees	Legs, Core, Cardio	Run in place lifting knees high, maintain pace. Perform for 45 seconds.
	(2) Plank with Shoulder Tap	Core, Shoulders, Triceps	In plank position, tap opposite shoulder with each hand. Perform for 45 seconds.
	(3) Jumping Jacks	Full Body, Cardio, Legs	Jump to spread legs and clap hands overhead. Perform for 45 seconds.
	(4) Skater Squat	Legs, Glutes, Core	Balance on one leg, squat, touch opposite hand to foot. Perform for 45 seconds.
121	**As many rounds as possible in 10 mins of:**		
	(1) Burpees (10 reps)	Full Body, Core, Legs	Jump, squat down, kick back into a push-up, return up. Perform 10 reps.
	(2) Russian Twists (20 reps)	Core, Obliques, Hip Flexors	Twist torso holding weight, seated on ground. Perform 20 reps.
	(3) Step-Ups (15 reps each leg)	Legs, Glutes, Core	Step onto a raised platform, alternate legs. Perform 15 reps each leg.
122	**50 seconds work, 10 seconds rest per exercise for 4 rounds:**		
	(1) High Knees	Legs, Core, Cardio	Run in place lifting knees high, maintain pace. Perform for 45 seconds.
	(2) Plank Jacks	Core, Shoulders, Cardio	Jump feet in and out while holding a plank position. Perform for 45 seconds.
	(3) Squat Jumps	Legs, Glutes, Cardio	Perform a squat then jump explosively. Perform for 45 seconds.
	(4) Bicycle Crunches	Core, Obliques, Hip Flexors	Lie down, alternate elbows to opposite knees cycling legs. Perform for 45 seconds.

Workout No.	Workout	Main Muscle Groups	Instructions
123	**Every minute on the minute for 20 mins:**		
	(1) Pull-Ups (5 reps)	Back, Biceps, Shoulders	Pull body up on bar, chin above hands. Perform 5 reps.
	(2) Side Lunges (10 reps each side)	Legs, Glutes, Core	Step to side into lunge, keep other leg straight. Perform 10 reps each side.
	(3) Fire Hydrant (15 reps each leg)	Glutes, Core, Hip Flexors	On hands and knees, lift leg to side, keep knee bent. Perform 15 reps each leg.
124	**As many rounds as possible in 12 mins:**		
	(1) Tuck Jumps (10 reps)	Legs, Core, Cardio	Jump high, tuck knees to chest mid-air. Perform 10 reps.
	(2) Donkey Kicks (10 reps each leg)	Glutes, Core, Hamstrings	On hands and knees, kick one leg back and up. Perform 10 reps each leg.
	(3) Jumping Jacks (20 reps)	Full Body, Cardio, Legs	Jump to spread legs and clap hands overhead. Perform 20 reps.
125	**10 Rounds for time:**		
	(1) Inchworm (10 reps)	Full Body, Core, Shoulders	Walk hands forward from standing, hold plank, walk back. Perform 10 reps.
	(2) Single Leg Dead Lift (10 reps each leg)	Hamstrings, Glutes, Core	Balance on one leg, hinge forward, extend free leg back. Perform 10 reps each leg.
	(3) Cross-Body Mountain Climbers (15 reps each side)	Core, Shoulders, Cardio	Bring knee towards opposite elbow while in plank position. Perform 15 reps each side.
126	**45 seconds work, 15 seconds rest per exercise for 8 rounds:**		
	(1) Jumping Jacks	Full Body, Cardio, Legs	Jump to spread legs and clap hands overhead. Perform for 45 seconds.
	(2) Crab Walk	Triceps, Core, Glutes	Walk backward on hands and feet, hips elevated. Perform for 45 seconds.
	(3) Flutter Kicks	Core, Hip Flexors, Lower Abs	Lie on back, alternately kick legs in small, rapid motion. Perform for 45 seconds.
	(4) Bird Dog	Core, Glutes, Shoulders	Extend opposite arm and leg, kneeling position. Perform for 45 seconds.
127	**As many rounds as possible in 10 mins of:**		
	(1) Plank to Push-Up (10 reps)	Core, Shoulders, Triceps	Alternate between plank and push-up positions. Perform 10 reps.
	(2) Box Jumps (15 reps)	Legs, Glutes, Core	Jump onto and off a box repeatedly, land softly. Perform 15 reps.
	(3) Bicycle Crunches (20 reps)	Core, Obliques, Hip Flexors	Lie down, alternate elbows to opposite knees cycling legs. Perform 20 reps.
128	**As many rounds as possible in 12 mins:**		
	(1) High Knees (30 seconds)	Legs, Core, Cardio	Run in place lifting knees high, maintain pace. Perform for 30 seconds.
	(2) Side-to-Side Push-Ups (10 reps each side)	Chest, Shoulders, Core	Shift side-to-side during push-ups, engages core. Perform 10 reps each side.
	(3) Jumping Jacks (30 seconds)	Full Body, Cardio, Legs	Jump to spread legs and clap hands overhead. Perform for 30 seconds.

Workout No.	Workout	Main Muscle Groups	Instructions
129	Every minute on the minute for 20 mins:		
	(1) Pull-Ups (5 reps)	Back, Biceps, Shoulders	Pull body up on bar, chin above hands. Perform 5 reps.
	(2) V-Ups (10 reps)	Core, Hip Flexors, Lower Abs	Lie back, lift legs and torso simultaneously, form 'V'. Perform 10 reps.
	(3) Step-Ups (15 reps each leg)	Legs, Glutes, Core	Step onto a raised platform, alternate legs. Perform 15 reps each leg.
130	45 seconds work, 15 seconds rest per exercise for 5 rounds:		
	(1) High Knees	Legs, Core, Cardio	Run in place lifting knees high, maintain pace. Perform for 45 seconds.
	(2) Plank with Shoulder Tap	Core, Shoulders, Triceps	In plank position, tap opposite shoulder with each hand. Perform for 45 seconds.
	(3) Squat Jumps	Legs, Glutes, Cardio	Perform a squat then jump explosively. Perform for 45 seconds.
	(4) Skater Squats	Legs, Glutes, Core	Balance on one leg, squat, touch opposite hand to foot. Perform for 45 seconds.
131	As many rounds as possible in 10 mins of:		
	(1) Burpees (15 reps)	Full Body, Core, Legs	Jump, squat down, kick back into a push-up, return up. Perform 15 reps.
	(2) Reverse Crunches (20 reps)	Core, Hip Flexors, Lower Abs	Lift hips off floor, knees towards chest. Perform 20 reps.
	(3) Glute Bridges (20 reps)	Glutes, Core, Hamstrings	Lift hips while lying on back, feet flat on ground. Perform 20 reps.
132	45 seconds work, 15 seconds rest per exercise for 4 rounds:		
	(1) High Knees	Legs, Core, Cardio	Run in place lifting knees high, maintain pace. Perform for 45 seconds.
	(2) Cross-Body Crunch	Core, Obliques, Hip Flexors	Touch opposite knee to elbow, lying down. Perform for 45 seconds.
	(3) Jumping Jacks	Full Body, Cardio, Legs	Jump to spread legs and clap hands overhead. Perform for 45 seconds.
	(4) Plank to Push-Up	Core, Shoulders, Triceps	Alternate between plank and push-up positions. Perform for 45 seconds.
133	Every minute on the minute for 21 mins:		
	(1) Pull-Ups (5 reps)	Back, Biceps, Shoulders	Pull body up on bar, chin above hands. Perform 5 reps.
	(2) Side Lunges (10 reps each side)	Legs, Glutes, Core	Step to side into lunge, keep other leg straight. Perform 10 reps each side.
	(3) Fire Hydrant (15 reps each leg)	Glutes, Core, Hip Flexors	On hands and knees, lift leg to side, keep knee bent. Perform 15 reps each leg.
134	As many rounds as possible in 12 mins:		
	(1) Tuck Jumps (10 reps)	Legs, Core, Cardio	Jump high, tuck knees to chest mid-air. Perform 10 reps.
	(2) Donkey Kicks (10 reps each leg)	Glutes, Core, Hamstrings	On hands and knees, kick one leg back and up. Perform 10 reps each leg.
	(3) Jumping Jacks (20 reps)	Full Body, Cardio, Legs	Jump to spread legs and clap hands overhead. Perform 20 reps.

Workout No.	Workout	Main Muscle Groups	Instructions
135	5 Rounds for time:		
	(1) Inchworm (10 reps)	Full Body, Core, Shoulders	Walk hands forward from standing, hold plank, walk back. Perform 10 reps.
	(2) Single Leg Dead Lift (10 reps each leg)	Hamstrings, Glutes, Core	Balance on one leg, hinge forward, extend free leg back. Perform 10 reps each leg.
	(3) Cross-Body Mountain Climbers (15 reps each side)	Core, Shoulders, Cardio	Bring knee towards opposite elbow while in plank position. Perform 15 reps each side.
136	50 seconds work, 10 seconds rest per exercise for 5 rounds:		
	(1) Jumping Jacks	Full Body, Cardio, Legs	Jump to spread legs and clap hands overhead. Perform for 45 seconds.
	(2) Crab Walk	Triceps, Core, Glutes	Walk backward on hands and feet, hips elevated. Perform for 45 seconds.
	(3) Flutter Kicks	Core, Hip Flexors, Lower Abs	Lie on back, alternately kick legs in small, rapid motion. Perform for 45 seconds.
	(4) Bird Dog	Core, Glutes, Shoulders	Extend opposite arm and leg, kneeling position. Perform for 45 seconds.
137	As many rounds as possible in 10 mins of:		
	(1) Squat Jumps (15 reps)	Legs, Glutes, Core	Perform a squat then jump explosively. Perform 15 reps.
	(2) Pike Push-Ups (10 reps)	Shoulders, Triceps, Core	Push-up with hips high, resembles downward dog pose. Perform 10 reps.
	(3) Bicycle Crunches (20 reps)	Core, Obliques, Hip Flexors	Lie down, alternate elbows to opposite knees cycling legs. Perform 20 reps.
138	As many rounds as possible in 15 mins:		
	(1) High Knees (30 seconds)	Legs, Core, Cardio	Run in place lifting knees high, maintain pace. Perform for 30 seconds.
	(2) Side-to-Side Push-Ups (10 reps each side)	Chest, Shoulders, Core	Shift side-to-side during push-ups, engages core. Perform 10 reps each side.
	(3) Jumping Jacks (30 seconds)	Full Body, Cardio, Legs	Jump to spread legs and clap hands overhead. Perform for 30 seconds.
139	Every minute on the minute for 20 mins:		
	(1) Pull-Ups (5 reps)	Back, Biceps, Shoulders	Pull body up on bar, chin above hands. Perform 5 reps.
	(2) V-Ups (10 reps)	Core, Hip Flexors, Lower Abs	Lie back, lift legs and torso simultaneously, form 'V'. Perform 10 reps.
	(3) Step-Ups (15 reps each leg)	Legs, Glutes, Core	Step onto a raised platform, alternate legs. Perform 15 reps each leg.
140	45 seconds work, 15 seconds rest per exercise for 8 rounds:		
	(1) High Knees	Legs, Core, Cardio	Run in place lifting knees high, maintain pace. Perform for 45 seconds.
	(2) Plank with Shoulder Tap	Core, Shoulders, Triceps	In plank position, tap opposite shoulder with each hand. Perform for 45 seconds.
	(3) Squat Jumps	Legs, Glutes, Cardio	Perform a squat then jump explosively. Perform for 45 seconds.
	(4) Skater Squats	Legs, Glutes, Core	Balance on one leg, squat, touch opposite hand to foot. Perform for 45 seconds.

Workout No.	Workout	Main Muscle Groups	Instructions
141	As many rounds as possible in 10 mins of:		
	(1) Box Jumps (15 reps)	Legs, Glutes, Core	Jump onto and off a box repeatedly, land softly. Perform 15 reps.
	(2) Side Plank (30 seconds each side)	Core, Shoulders, Obliques	Support body on one arm, side facing ground. Hold for 30 seconds each side.
	(3) Walking Lunges (15 reps each leg)	Legs, Glutes, Core	Step forward into a lunge, move forward alternating legs. Perform 15 reps each leg.
142	45 seconds work, 15 seconds rest per exercise for 4 rounds:		
	(1) High Knees	Legs, Core, Cardio	Run in place lifting knees high, maintain pace. Perform for 45 seconds.
	(2) Cross-Body Crunch	Core, Obliques, Hip Flexors	Touch opposite knee to elbow, lying down. Perform for 45 seconds.
	(3) Jumping Jacks	Full Body, Cardio, Legs	Jump to spread legs and clap hands overhead. Perform for 45 seconds.
	(4) Plank Rotation	Core, Shoulders, Obliques	Rotate body in plank, extend arm upward, switch sides. Perform for 45 seconds.
143	Every minute on the minute for 20 mins:		
	(1) Pull-Ups (5 reps)	Back, Biceps, Shoulders	Pull body up on bar, chin above hands. Perform 5 reps.
	(2) Glute Bridge (15 reps)	Glutes, Core, Hamstrings	Lift hips while lying on back, feet flat on ground. Perform 15 reps.
	(3) Side Lunges (10 reps each side)	Legs, Glutes, Core	Step to side into lunge, keep other leg straight. Perform 10 reps each side.
144	As many rounds as possible in 12 mins:		
	(1) Tuck Jumps (10 reps)	Legs, Core, Cardio	Jump high, tuck knees to chest mid-air. Perform 10 reps.
	(2) Donkey Kicks (10 reps each leg)	Glutes, Core, Hamstrings	On hands and knees, kick one leg back and up. Perform 10 reps each leg.
	(3) Jumping Jacks (20 reps)	Full Body, Cardio, Legs	Jump to spread legs and clap hands overhead. Perform 20 reps.
145	6 Rounds for time:		
	(1) Inchworm (10 reps)	Full Body, Core, Shoulders	Walk hands forward from standing, hold plank, walk back. Perform 10 reps.
	(2) Single Leg Dead Lift (10 reps each leg)	Hamstrings, Glutes, Core	Balance on one leg, hinge forward, extend free leg back. Perform 10 reps each leg.
	(3) Cross-Body Mountain Climbers (15 reps each side)	Core, Shoulders, Cardio	Bring knee towards opposite elbow while in plank position. Perform 15 reps each side.
146	45 seconds work, 15 seconds rest per exercise for 5 rounds:		
	(1) Jumping Jacks	Full Body, Cardio, Legs	Jump to spread legs and clap hands overhead. Perform for 45 seconds.
	(2) Crab Walk	Triceps, Core, Glutes	Walk backward on hands and feet, hips elevated. Perform for 45 seconds.
	(3) Flutter Kicks	Core, Hip Flexors, Lower Abs	Lie on back, alternately kick legs in small, rapid motion. Perform for 45 seconds.
	(4) Bird Dog	Core, Glutes, Shoulders	Extend opposite arm and leg, kneeling position. Perform for 45 seconds.

Workout No.	Workout	Main Muscle Groups	Instructions
147	**As many rounds as possible in 10 mins of:**		
	(1) Squat Jumps (15 reps)	Legs, Glutes, Core	Perform a squat then jump explosively. Perform 15 reps.
	(2) Pike Push-Ups (10 reps)	Shoulders, Triceps, Core	Push-up with hips high, resembles downward dog pose. Perform 10 reps.
	(3) Bicycle Crunches (20 reps)	Core, Obliques, Hip Flexors	Lie down, alternate elbows to opposite knees cycling legs. Perform 20 reps.
148	**As many rounds as possible in 12 mins:**		
	(1) High Knees (30 seconds)	Legs, Core, Cardio	Run in place lifting knees high, maintain pace. Perform for 30 seconds.
	(2) Side-to-Side Push-Ups (10 reps each side)	Chest, Shoulders, Core	Shift side-to-side during push-ups, engages core. Perform 10 reps each side.
	(3) Jumping Jacks (30 seconds)	Full Body, Cardio, Legs	Jump to spread legs and clap hands overhead. Perform for 30 seconds.
149	**Every minute on the minute for 20 mins:**		
	(1) Pull-Ups (5 reps)	Back, Biceps, Shoulders	Pull body up on bar, chin above hands. Perform 5 reps.
	(2) V-Ups (10 reps)	Core, Hip Flexors, Lower Abs	Lie back, lift legs and torso simultaneously, form 'V'. Perform 10 reps.
	(3) Step-Ups (15 reps each leg)	Legs, Glutes, Core	Step onto a raised platform, alternate legs. Perform 15 reps each leg.
150	**30 seconds work, 30 seconds rest per exercise for 9 rounds:**		
	(1) High Knees	Legs, Core, Cardio	Run in place lifting knees high, maintain pace. Perform for 45 seconds.
	(2) Plank with Shoulder Tap	Core, Shoulders, Triceps	In plank position, tap opposite shoulder with each hand. Perform for 45 seconds.
	(3) Squat Jumps	Legs, Glutes, Cardio	Perform a squat then jump explosively. Perform for 45 seconds.
	(4) Skater Squats	Legs, Glutes, Core	Balance on one leg, squat, touch opposite hand to foot. Perform for 45 seconds.
151	**As many rounds as possible in 10 mins of:**		
	(1) Burpees (10 reps)	Full Body, Core, Legs	Jump, squat down, kick back into a push-up, return up. Perform 10 reps.
	(2) Russian Twists (20 reps)	Core, Obliques, Hip Flexors	Twist torso holding weight, seated on ground. Perform 20 reps.
	(3) Step-Ups (15 reps each leg)	Legs, Glutes, Core	Step onto a raised platform, alternate legs. Perform 15 reps each leg.
152	**45 seconds work, 15 seconds rest per exercise for 4 rounds:**		
	(1) High Knees	Legs, Core, Cardio	Run in place lifting knees high, maintain pace. Perform for 45 seconds.
	(2) Plank Jacks	Core, Shoulders, Cardio	Jump feet in and out while holding a plank position. Perform for 45 seconds.
	(3) Squat Jumps	Legs, Glutes, Cardio	Perform a squat then jump explosively. Perform for 45 seconds.
	(4) Bicycle Crunches	Core, Obliques, Hip Flexors	Lie down, alternate elbows to opposite knees cycling legs. Perform for 45 seconds.

Workout No.	Workout	Main Muscle Groups	Instructions
153	**Every minute on the minute for 20 mins:**		
	(1) Pull-Ups (5 reps)	Back, Biceps, Shoulders	Pull body up on bar, chin above hands. Perform 5 reps.
	(2) Side Lunges (10 reps each side)	Legs, Glutes, Core	Step to side into lunge, keep other leg straight. Perform 10 reps each side.
	(3) Fire Hydrant (15 reps each leg)	Glutes, Core, Hip Flexors	On hands and knees, lift leg to side, keep knee bent. Perform 15 reps each leg.
154	**As many rounds as possible in 12 mins:**		
	(1) Tuck Jumps (10 reps)	Legs, Core, Cardio	Jump high, tuck knees to chest mid-air. Perform 10 reps.
	(2) Donkey Kicks (10 reps each leg)	Glutes, Core, Hamstrings	On hands and knees, kick one leg back and up. Perform 10 reps each leg.
	(3) Jumping Jacks (20 reps)	Full Body, Cardio, Legs	Jump to spread legs and clap hands overhead. Perform 20 reps.
155	**5 Rounds for time:**		
	(1) Inchworm (10 reps)	Full Body, Core, Shoulders	Walk hands forward from standing, hold plank, walk back. Perform 10 reps.
	(2) Single Leg Dead Lift (10 reps each leg)	Hamstrings, Glutes, Core	Balance on one leg, hinge forward, extend free leg back. Perform 10 reps each leg.
	(3) Cross-Body Mountain Climbers (15 reps each side)	Core, Shoulders, Cardio	Bring knee towards opposite elbow while in plank position. Perform 15 reps each side.
156	**50 seconds work, 10 seconds rest per exercise for 5 rounds:**		
	(1) Jumping Jacks	Full Body, Cardio, Legs	Jump to spread legs and clap hands overhead. Perform for 45 seconds.
	(2) Crab Walk	Triceps, Core, Glutes	Walk backward on hands and feet, hips elevated. Perform for 45 seconds.
	(3) Flutter Kicks	Core, Hip Flexors, Lower Abs	Lie on back, alternately kick legs in small, rapid motion. Perform for 45 seconds.
	(4) Bird Dog	Core, Glutes, Shoulders	Extend opposite arm and leg, kneeling position. Perform for 45 seconds.
157	**As many rounds as possible in 10 mins of:**		
	(1) Plank to Push-Up (10 reps)	Core, Shoulders, Triceps	Alternate between plank and push-up positions. Perform 10 reps.
	(2) Box Jumps (15 reps)	Legs, Glutes, Core	Jump onto and off a box repeatedly, land softly. Perform 15 reps.
	(3) Bicycle Crunches (20 reps)	Core, Obliques, Hip Flexors	Lie down, alternate elbows to opposite knees cycling legs. Perform 20 reps.
158	**As many rounds as possible in 12 mins:**		
	(1) High Knees (30 seconds)	Legs, Core, Cardio	Run in place lifting knees high, maintain pace. Perform for 30 seconds.
	(2) Side-to-Side Push-Ups (10 reps each side)	Chest, Shoulders, Core	Shift side-to-side during push-ups, engages core. Perform 10 reps each side.
	(3) Jumping Jacks (30 seconds)	Full Body, Cardio, Legs	Jump to spread legs and clap hands overhead. Perform for 30 seconds.

Workout No.	Workout		Main Muscle Groups	Instructions
159	Every minute on the minute for 20 mins:			
	(1)	Pull-Ups (5 reps)	Back, Biceps, Shoulders	Pull body up on bar, chin above hands. Perform 5 reps.
	(2)	V-Ups (10 reps)	Core, Hip Flexors, Lower Abs	Lie back, lift legs and torso simultaneously, form 'V'. Perform 10 reps.
	(3)	Step-Ups (15 reps each leg)	Legs, Glutes, Core	Step onto a raised platform, alternate legs. Perform 15 reps each leg.
160	45 seconds work, 15 seconds rest per exercise for 5 rounds:			
	(1)	High Knees	Legs, Core, Cardio	Run in place lifting knees high, maintain pace. Perform for 45 seconds.
	(2)	Plank with Shoulder Tap	Core, Shoulders, Triceps	In plank position, tap opposite shoulder with each hand. Perform for 45 seconds.
	(3)	Squat Jumps	Legs, Glutes, Cardio	Perform a squat then jump explosively. Perform for 45 seconds.
	(4)	Skater Squats	Legs, Glutes, Core	Balance on one leg, squat, touch opposite hand to foot. Perform for 45 seconds.
161	As many rounds as possible in 10 mins of:			
	(1)	Jumping Jacks (20 reps)	Full Body, Cardio, Legs	Jump to spread legs and clap hands overhead. Perform 20 reps.
	(2)	Pull-Ups (5 reps)	Back, Biceps, Shoulders	Pull body up on bar, chin above hands. Perform 5 reps.
	(3)	Fire Hydrant (15 reps each leg)	Glutes, Core, Hip Flexors	On hands and knees, lift leg to side, keep knee bent. Perform 15 reps each leg.
162	45 seconds work, 15 seconds rest per exercise for 4 rounds:			
	(1)	High Knees	Legs, Core, Cardio	Run in place lifting knees high, maintain pace. Perform for 45 seconds.
	(2)	Cross-Body Crunch	Core, Obliques, Hip Flexors	Touch opposite knee to elbow, lying down. Perform for 45 seconds.
	(3)	Squat Jumps	Legs, Glutes, Cardio	Perform a squat then jump explosively. Perform for 45 seconds.
	(4)	Plank to Push-Up	Core, Shoulders, Triceps	Alternate between plank and push-up positions. Perform for 45 seconds.
163	Every minute on the minute for 20 mins:			
	(1)	Pull-Ups (5 reps)	Back, Biceps, Shoulders	Pull body up on bar, chin above hands. Perform 5 reps.
	(2)	Glute Bridge (15 reps)	Glutes, Core, Hamstrings	Lift hips while lying on back, feet flat on ground. Perform 15 reps.
	(3)	Side Lunges (10 reps each side)	Legs, Glutes, Core	Step to side into lunge, keep other leg straight. Perform 10 reps each side.
164	As many rounds as possible in 12 mins:			
	(1)	Tuck Jumps (10 reps)	Legs, Core, Cardio	Jump high, tuck knees to chest mid-air. Perform 10 reps.
	(2)	Donkey Kicks (10 reps each leg)	Glutes, Core, Hamstrings	On hands and knees, kick one leg back and up. Perform 10 reps each leg.
	(3)	Mountain Climbers (20 reps)	Core, Legs, Shoulders	Run in place in plank position, drive knees to chest. Perform 20 reps.

Workout No.		Workout	Main Muscle Groups	Instructions
165		**5 Rounds for time:**		
	(1)	Inchworm (10 reps)	Full Body, Core, Shoulders	Walk hands forward from standing, hold plank, walk back. Perform 10 reps.
	(2)	Single Leg Dead Lift (10 reps each leg)	Hamstrings, Glutes, Core	Balance on one leg, hinge forward, extend free leg back. Perform 10 reps each leg.
	(3)	Cross-Body Mountain Climbers (15 reps each side)	Core, Shoulders, Cardio	Bring knee towards opposite elbow while in plank position. Perform 15 reps each side.
166		**45 seconds work, 15 seconds rest per exercise for 8 rounds:**		
	(1)	Jumping Jacks	Full Body, Cardio, Legs	Jump to spread legs and clap hands overhead. Perform for 45 seconds.
	(2)	Crab Walk	Triceps, Core, Glutes	Walk backward on hands and feet, hips elevated. Perform for 45 seconds.
	(3)	Flutter Kicks	Core, Hip Flexors, Lower Abs	Lie on back, alternately kick legs in small, rapid motion. Perform for 45 seconds.
	(4)	Bird Dog	Core, Glutes, Shoulders	Extend opposite arm and leg, kneeling position. Perform for 45 seconds.
167		**As many rounds as possible in 10 mins of:**		
	(1)	Squat Jumps (15 reps)	Legs, Glutes, Core	Perform a squat then jump explosively. Perform 15 reps.
	(2)	Pike Push-Ups (10 reps)	Shoulders, Triceps, Core	Push-up with hips high, resembles downward dog pose. Perform 10 reps.
	(3)	Bicycle Crunches (20 reps)	Core, Obliques, Hip Flexors	Lie down, alternate elbows to opposite knees cycling legs. Perform 20 reps.
168		**As many rounds as possible in 12 mins:**		
	(1)	High Knees (30 seconds)	Legs, Core, Cardio	Run in place lifting knees high, maintain pace. Perform for 30 seconds.
	(2)	Side-to-Side Push-Ups (10 reps each side)	Chest, Shoulders, Core	Shift side-to-side during push-ups, engages core. Perform 10 reps each side.
	(3)	Jumping Jacks (30 seconds)	Full Body, Cardio, Legs	Jump to spread legs and clap hands overhead. Perform for 30 seconds.
169		**Every minute on the minute for 20 mins:**		
	(1)	Pull-Ups (5 reps)	Back, Biceps, Shoulders	Pull body up on bar, chin above hands. Perform 5 reps.
	(2)	V-Ups (10 reps)	Core, Hip Flexors, Lower Abs	Lie back, lift legs and torso simultaneously, form 'V'. Perform 10 reps.
	(3)	Step-Ups (15 reps each leg)	Legs, Glutes, Core	Step onto a raised platform, alternate legs. Perform 15 reps each leg.
170		**45 seconds work, 15 seconds rest per exercise for 4 rounds:**		
	(1)	High Knees	Legs, Core, Cardio	Run in place lifting knees high, maintain pace. Perform for 45 seconds.
	(2)	Plank with Shoulder Tap	Core, Shoulders, Triceps	In plank position, tap opposite shoulder with each hand. Perform for 45 seconds.
	(3)	Squat Jumps	Legs, Glutes, Cardio	Perform a squat then jump explosively. Perform for 45 seconds.
	(4)	Skater Squats	Legs, Glutes, Core	Balance on one leg, squat, touch opposite hand to foot. Perform for 45 seconds.

Workout No.	Workout	Main Muscle Groups	Instructions
171	**As many rounds as possible in 10 mins of:**		
	(1) Box Jumps (15 reps)	Legs, Glutes, Core	Jump onto and off a box repeatedly, land softly. Perform 15 reps.
	(2) Plank with Shoulder Tap (20 reps)	Core, Shoulders, Triceps	In plank position, tap opposite shoulder with each hand. Perform 20 reps.
	(3) Walking Lunges (15 reps each leg)	Legs, Glutes, Core	Step forward into a lunge, move forward alternating legs. Perform 15 reps each leg.
172	**45 seconds work, 15 seconds rest per exercise for 5 rounds:**		
	(1) High Knees	Legs, Core, Cardio	Run in place lifting knees high, maintain pace. Perform for 45 seconds.
	(2) Cross-Body Crunch	Core, Obliques, Hip Flexors	Touch opposite knee to elbow, lying down. Perform for 45 seconds.
	(3) Squat Jumps	Legs, Glutes, Cardio	Perform a squat then jump explosively. Perform for 45 seconds.
	(4) Bird Dog	Core, Glutes, Shoulders	Extend opposite arm and leg, kneeling position. Perform for 45 seconds.
173	**Every minute on the minute for 20 mins:**		
	(1) Pull-Ups (5 reps)	Back, Biceps, Shoulders	Pull body up on bar, chin above hands. Perform 5 reps.
	(2) Glute Bridge (15 reps)	Glutes, Core, Hamstrings	Lift hips while lying on back, feet flat on ground. Perform 15 reps.
	(3) Side Lunges (10 reps each side)	Legs, Glutes, Core	Step to side into lunge, keep other leg straight. Perform 10 reps each side.
174	**As many rounds as possible in 12 mins:**		
	(1) Tuck Jumps (10 reps)	Legs, Core, Cardio	Jump high, tuck knees to chest mid-air. Perform 10 reps.
	(2) Donkey Kicks (10 reps each leg)	Glutes, Core, Hamstrings	On hands and knees, kick one leg back and up. Perform 10 reps each leg.
	(3) Jumping Jacks (20 reps)	Full Body, Cardio, Legs	Jump to spread legs and clap hands overhead. Perform 20 reps.
175	**5 Rounds for time:**		
	(1) Inchworm (10 reps)	Full Body, Core, Shoulders	Walk hands forward from standing, hold plank, walk back. Perform 10 reps.
	(2) Single Leg Dead Lift (10 reps each leg)	Hamstrings, Glutes, Core	Balance on one leg, hinge forward, extend free leg back. Perform 10 reps each leg.
	(3) Cross-Body Mountain Climbers (15 reps each side)	Core, Shoulders, Cardio	Bring knee towards opposite elbow while in plank position. Perform 15 reps each side.
176	**45 seconds work, 15 seconds rest per exercise for 4 rounds:**		
	(1) Jumping Jacks	Full Body, Cardio, Legs	Jump to spread legs and clap hands overhead. Perform for 45 seconds.
	(2) Crab Walk	Triceps, Core, Glutes	Walk backward on hands and feet, hips elevated. Perform for 45 seconds.
	(3) Flutter Kicks	Core, Hip Flexors, Lower Abs	Lie on back, alternately kick legs in small, rapid motion. Perform for 45 seconds.
	(4) Bear Crawl	Full Body, Core, Shoulders	Crawl forward on all fours, hips down, move quickly. Perform for 45 seconds.

Workout No.	Workout	Main Muscle Groups	Instructions
177	As many rounds as possible in 10 mins of:		
	(1) Squat Jumps (15 reps)	Legs, Glutes, Core	Perform a squat then jump explosively. Perform 15 reps.
	(2) Pike Push-Ups (10 reps)	Shoulders, Triceps, Core	Push-up with hips high, resembles downward dog pose. Perform 10 reps.
	(3) Bicycle Crunches (20 reps)	Core, Obliques, Hip Flexors	Lie down, alternate elbows to opposite knees cycling legs. Perform 20 reps.
178	As many rounds as possible in 12 mins:		
	(1) High Knees (30 seconds)	Legs, Core, Cardio	Run in place lifting knees high, maintain pace. Perform for 30 seconds.
	(2) Side-to-Side Push-Ups (10 reps each side)	Chest, Shoulders, Core	Shift side-to-side during push-ups, engages core. Perform 10 reps each side.
	(3) Jumping Jacks (30 seconds)	Full Body, Cardio, Legs	Jump to spread legs and clap hands overhead. Perform for 30 seconds.
179	Every minute on the minute for 20 mins:		
	(1) Pull-Ups (5 reps)	Back, Biceps, Shoulders	Pull body up on bar, chin above hands. Perform 5 reps.
	(2) V-Ups (10 reps)	Core, Hip Flexors, Lower Abs	Lie back, lift legs and torso simultaneously, form 'V'. Perform 10 reps.
	(3) Step-Ups (15 reps each leg)	Legs, Glutes, Core	Step onto a raised platform, alternate legs. Perform 15 reps each leg.
180	50 seconds work, 10 seconds rest per exercise for 5 rounds:		
	(1) High Knees	Legs, Core, Cardio	Run in place lifting knees high, maintain pace. Perform for 45 seconds.
	(2) Plank with Shoulder Tap	Core, Shoulders, Triceps	In plank position, tap opposite shoulder with each hand. Perform for 45 seconds.
	(3) Mountain Climbers	Core, Legs, Shoulders	Run in place in plank position, drive knees to chest. Perform for 45 seconds.
	(4) Skater Squats	Legs, Glutes, Core	Balance on one leg, squat, touch opposite hand to foot. Perform for 45 seconds.
181	As many rounds as possible in 10 mins of:		
	(1) Burpees (10 reps)	Full Body, Core, Legs	Jump, squat down, kick back into a push-up, return up. Perform 10 reps.
	(2) Lunge (15 reps each leg)	Legs, Glutes, Core	Step forward, lower hips to drop knee to ground. Perform 15 reps each leg.
	(3) Plank (1 min)	Core, Shoulders, Back	Hold body straight on elbows, maintain line. Hold for 1 minute.
182	45 seconds work, 15 seconds rest per exercise for 4 rounds:		
	(1) High Knees	Legs, Core, Cardio	Run in place lifting knees high, maintain pace. Perform for 45 seconds.
	(2) Russian Twists	Core, Obliques, Hip Flexors	Twist torso holding weight, seated on ground. Perform for 45 seconds.
	(3) Jumping Jacks	Full Body, Cardio, Legs	Jump to spread legs and clap hands overhead. Perform for 45 seconds.
	(4) Flutter Kicks	Core, Hip Flexors, Lower Abs	Lie on back, alternately kick legs in small, rapid motion. Perform for 45 seconds.

Workout No.	Workout	Main Muscle Groups	Instructions
183	**Every minute on the minute for 20 mins:**		
	(1) Pull-Ups (5 reps)	Back, Biceps, Shoulders	Pull body up on bar, chin above hands. Perform 5 reps.
	(2) V-Ups (10 reps)	Core, Hip Flexors, Lower Abs	Lie back, lift legs and torso simultaneously, form 'V'. Perform 10 reps.
	(3) Donkey Kicks (15 reps each leg)	Glutes, Core, Hamstrings	On hands and knees, kick one leg back and up. Perform 15 reps each leg.
184	**As many rounds as possible in 12 mins:**		
	(1) Tuck Jumps (10 reps)	Legs, Core, Cardio	Jump high, tuck knees to chest mid-air. Perform 10 reps.
	(2) Bird Dog (10 reps each side)	Core, Glutes, Shoulders	Extend opposite arm and leg, kneeling position. Perform 10 reps each side.
	(3) Jumping Jacks (20 reps)	Full Body, Cardio, Legs	Jump to spread legs and clap hands overhead. Perform 20 reps.
185	**5 Rounds for time:**		
	(1) Inchworm (10 reps)	Full Body, Core, Shoulders	Walk hands forward from standing, hold plank, walk back. Perform 10 reps.
	(2) Single Leg Dead Lift (10 reps each leg)	Hamstrings, Glutes, Core	Balance on one leg, hinge forward, extend free leg back. Perform 10 reps each leg.
	(3) Cross-Body Mountain Climbers (15 reps each side)	Core, Shoulders, Cardio	Bring knee towards opposite elbow while in plank position. Perform 15 reps each side.
186	**45 seconds work, 15 seconds rest per exercise for 4 rounds:**		
	(1) Jumping Jacks	Full Body, Cardio, Legs	Jump to spread legs and clap hands overhead. Perform for 45 seconds.
	(2) Crab Walk	Triceps, Core, Glutes	Walk backward on hands and feet, hips elevated. Perform for 45 seconds.
	(3) Side Plank (each side)	Core, Obliques, Shoulders	Support body on one arm, side facing ground. Hold for 45 seconds each side.
	(4) High Knees	Legs, Core, Cardio	Run in place lifting knees high, maintain pace. Perform for 45 seconds.
187	**As many rounds as possible in 10 mins of:**		
	(1) Plank to Push-Up (10 reps)	Core, Shoulders, Triceps	Alternate between plank and push-up positions. Perform 10 reps.
	(2) Box Jumps (15 reps)	Legs, Glutes, Core	Jump onto and off a box repeatedly, land softly. Perform 15 reps.
	(3) Bicycle Crunches (20 reps)	Core, Obliques, Hip Flexors	Lie down, alternate elbows to opposite knees cycling legs. Perform 20 reps.
188	**As many rounds as possible in 12 mins:**		
	(1) High Knees (30 seconds)	Legs, Core, Cardio	Run in place lifting knees high, maintain pace. Perform for 30 seconds.
	(2) Side-to-Side Push-Ups (10 reps each side)	Chest, Shoulders, Core	Shift side-to-side during push-ups, engages core. Perform 10 reps each side.
	(3) Jumping Jacks (30 seconds)	Full Body, Cardio, Legs	Jump to spread legs and clap hands overhead. Perform for 30 seconds.

Workout No.	Workout	Main Muscle Groups	Instructions
189	**Every minute on the minute for 20 mins:**		
	(1) Pull-Ups (5 reps)	Back, Biceps, Shoulders	Pull body up on bar, chin above hands. Perform 5 reps.
	(2) Glute Bridge (15 reps)	Glutes, Core, Hamstrings	Lift hips while lying on back, feet flat on ground. Perform 15 reps.
	(3) Fire Hydrant (15 reps each leg)	Glutes, Core, Hip Flexors	On hands and knees, lift leg to side, keep knee bent. Perform 15 reps each leg.
190	**50 seconds work, 10 seconds rest per exercise for 4 rounds:**		
	(1) High Knees	Legs, Core, Cardio	Run in place lifting knees high, maintain pace. Perform for 45 seconds.
	(2) Plank with Shoulder Tap	Core, Shoulders, Triceps	In plank position, tap opposite shoulder with each hand. Perform for 45 seconds.
	(3) Squat Jumps	Legs, Glutes, Cardio	Perform a squat then jump explosively. Perform for 45 seconds.
	(4) Skater Squats	Legs, Glutes, Core	Balance on one leg, squat, touch opposite hand to foot. Perform for 45 seconds.
	(5) Side Lunges (45 seconds on, 15 seconds off x 4 rounds)	Legs, Glutes, Core	Step to side into lunge, keep other leg straight. Repeat on the other side.
191	**As many rounds as possible in 10 mins of:**		
	(1) Burpees (10 reps)	Full Body, Core, Legs	Jump, squat down, kick back into a push-up, return up. Perform 10 reps.
	(2) Side Plank (30 seconds each side)	Core, Shoulders, Obliques	Support body on one arm, side facing ground. Hold for 30 seconds each side.
	(3) Step-Ups (15 reps each leg)	Legs, Glutes, Core	Step onto a raised platform, alternate legs. Perform 15 reps each leg.
192	**45 seconds work, 15 seconds rest per exercise for 4 rounds:**		
	(1) High Knees	Legs, Core, Cardio	Run in place lifting knees high, maintain pace. Perform for 45 seconds.
	(2) Cross-Body Crunch	Core, Obliques, Hip Flexors	Touch opposite knee to elbow, lying down. Perform for 45 seconds.
	(3) Jumping Jacks	Full Body, Cardio, Legs	Jump to spread legs and clap hands overhead. Perform for 45 seconds.
	(4) Bear Crawl	Full Body, Core, Shoulders	Crawl forward on all fours, hips down, move quickly. Perform for 45 seconds.
193	**Every minute on the minute for 20 mins:**		
	(1) Pull-Ups (5 reps)	Back, Biceps, Shoulders	Pull body up on bar, chin above hands. Perform 5 reps.
	(2) Glute Bridge (15 reps)	Glutes, Core, Hamstrings	Lift hips while lying on back, feet flat on ground. Perform 15 reps.
	(3) Side Lunges (10 reps each side)	Legs, Glutes, Core	Step to side into lunge, keep other leg straight. Perform 10 reps each side.

Workout No.		Workout	Main Muscle Groups	Instructions
194		**As many rounds as possible in 12 mins:**		
	(1)	Tuck Jumps (10 reps)	Legs, Core, Cardio	Jump high, tuck knees to chest mid-air. Perform 10 reps.
	(2)	Donkey Kicks (10 reps each leg)	Glutes, Core, Hamstrings	On hands and knees, kick one leg back and up. Perform 10 reps each leg.
	(3)	Mountain Climbers (20 reps)	Core, Legs, Shoulders	Run in place in plank position, drive knees to chest. Perform 20 reps.
195		**5 Rounds for time:**		
	(1)	Inchworm (10 reps)	Full Body, Core, Shoulders	Walk hands forward from standing, hold plank, walk back. Perform 10 reps.
	(2)	Single Leg Dead Lift (10 reps each leg)	Hamstrings, Glutes, Core	Balance on one leg, hinge forward, extend free leg back. Perform 10 reps each leg.
	(3)	Cross-Body Mountain Climbers (15 reps each side)	Core, Shoulders, Cardio	Bring knee towards opposite elbow while in plank position. Perform 15 reps each side.
196		**45 seconds work, 15 seconds rest per exercise for 4 rounds:**		
	(1)	Jumping Jacks	Full Body, Cardio, Legs	Jump to spread legs and clap hands overhead. Perform for 45 seconds.
	(2)	Crab Walk	Triceps, Core, Glutes	Walk backward on hands and feet, hips elevated. Perform for 45 seconds.
	(3)	Flutter Kicks	Core, Hip Flexors, Lower Abs	Lie on back, alternately kick legs in small, rapid motion. Perform for 45 seconds.
	(4)	Bird Dog	Core, Glutes, Shoulders	Extend opposite arm and leg, kneeling position. Perform for 45 seconds.
197		**As many rounds as possible in 10 mins of:**		
	(1)	Squat Jumps (15 reps)	Legs, Glutes, Core	Perform a squat then jump explosively. Perform 15 reps.
	(2)	Pike Push-Ups (10 reps)	Shoulders, Triceps, Core	Push-up with hips high, resembles downward dog pose. Perform 10 reps.
	(3)	Bicycle Crunches (20 reps)	Core, Obliques, Hip Flexors	Lie down, alternate elbows to opposite knees cycling legs. Perform 20 reps.
198		**As many rounds as possible in 12 mins:**		
	(1)	High Knees (30 seconds)	Legs, Core, Cardio	Run in place lifting knees high, maintain pace. Perform for 30 seconds.
	(2)	Side-to-Side Push-Ups (10 reps each side)	Chest, Shoulders, Core	Shift side-to-side during push-ups, engages core. Perform 10 reps each side.
	(3)	Jumping Jacks (30 seconds)	Full Body, Cardio, Legs	Jump to spread legs and clap hands overhead. Perform for 30 seconds.
199		**Every minute on the minute for 20 mins:**		
	(1)	Pull-Ups (5 reps)	Back, Biceps, Shoulders	Pull body up on bar, chin above hands. Perform 5 reps.
	(2)	V-Ups (10 reps)	Core, Hip Flexors, Lower Abs	Lie back, lift legs and torso simultaneously, form 'V'. Perform 10 reps.
	(3)	Step-Ups (15 reps each leg)	Legs, Glutes, Core	Step onto a raised platform, alternate legs. Perform 15 reps each leg.

Workout No.	Workout	Main Muscle Groups	Instructions
200	**40 seconds work, 20 seconds rest per exercise for 5 rounds:**		
	(1) High Knees	Legs, Core, Cardio	Run in place lifting knees high, maintain pace. Perform for 45 seconds.
	(2) Plank with Shoulder Tap	Core, Shoulders, Triceps	In plank position, tap opposite shoulder with each hand. Perform for 45 seconds.
	(3) Squat Jumps	Legs, Glutes, Cardio	Perform a squat then jump explosively. Perform for 45 seconds.
	(4) Skater Squats	Legs, Glutes, Core	Balance on one leg, squat, touch opposite hand to foot. Perform for 45 seconds.
201	**As many rounds as possible in 10 mins of:**		
	(1) Burpees (10 reps)	Full Body, Core, Legs	Jump, squat down, kick back into a push-up, return up. Perform 10 reps.
	(2) Reverse Crunch (15 reps)	Core, Hip Flexors, Lower Abs	Lift hips off floor, knees towards chest. Perform 15 reps.
	(3) Fire Hydrant (15 reps each leg)	Glutes, Core, Hip Flexors	On hands and knees, lift leg to side, keep knee bent. Perform 15 reps each leg.
202	**45 seconds work, 15 seconds rest per exercise for 4 rounds:**		
	(1) High Knees	Legs, Core, Cardio	Run in place lifting knees high, maintain pace. Perform for 45 seconds.
	(2) Plank with Shoulder Tap	Core, Shoulders, Triceps	In plank position, tap opposite shoulder with each hand. Perform for 45 seconds.
	(3) Jumping Jacks	Full Body, Cardio, Legs	Jump to spread legs and clap hands overhead. Perform for 45 seconds.
	(4) Russian Twists	Core, Obliques, Hip Flexors	Twist torso holding weight, seated on ground. Perform for 45 seconds.
203	**Every minute on the minute for 20 mins:**		
	(1) Pull-Ups (5 reps)	Back, Biceps, Shoulders	Pull body up on bar, chin above hands. Perform 5 reps.
	(2) V-Ups (10 reps)	Core, Hip Flexors, Lower Abs	Lie back, lift legs and torso simultaneously, form 'V'. Perform 10 reps.
	(3) Glute Bridge (15 reps)	Glutes, Core, Hamstrings	Lift hips while lying on back, feet flat on ground. Perform 15 reps.
204	**As many rounds as possible in 12 mins:**		
	(1) Tuck Jumps (10 reps)	Legs, Core, Cardio	Jump high, tuck knees to chest mid-air. Perform 10 reps.
	(2) Side Plank (30 seconds each side)	Core, Shoulders, Obliques	Support body on one arm, side facing ground. Hold for 30 seconds each side.
	(3) Mountain Climbers (20 reps)	Core, Legs, Shoulders	Run in place in plank position, drive knees to chest. Perform 20 reps.
205	**5 Rounds for time:**		
	(1) Inchworm (10 reps)	Full Body, Core, Shoulders	Walk hands forward from standing, hold plank, walk back. Perform 10 reps.
	(2) Single Leg Dead Lift (10 reps each leg)	Hamstrings, Glutes, Core	Balance on one leg, hinge forward, extend free leg back. Perform 10 reps each leg.
	(3) Cross-Body Mountain Climbers (15 reps each side)	Core, Shoulders, Cardio	Bring knee towards opposite elbow while in plank position. Perform 15 reps each side.

Workout No.	Workout	Main Muscle Groups	Instructions
206	45 seconds work, 15 seconds rest per exercise for 5 rounds:		
	(1) Jumping Jacks	Full Body, Cardio, Legs	Jump to spread legs and clap hands overhead. Perform for 45 seconds.
	(2) Crab Walk	Triceps, Core, Glutes	Walk backward on hands and feet, hips elevated. Perform for 45 seconds.
	(3) Flutter Kicks	Core, Hip Flexors, Lower Abs	Lie on back, alternately kick legs in small, rapid motion. Perform for 45 seconds.
	(4) Bird Dog	Core, Glutes, Shoulders	Extend opposite arm and leg, kneeling position. Perform for 45 seconds.
207	As many rounds as possible in 10 mins of:		
	(1) Squat Jumps (15 reps)	Legs, Glutes, Core	Perform a squat then jump explosively. Perform 15 reps.
	(2) Pike Push-Ups (10 reps)	Shoulders, Triceps, Core	Push-up with hips high, resembles downward dog pose. Perform 10 reps.
	(3) Bicycle Crunches (20 reps)	Core, Obliques, Hip Flexors	Lie down, alternate elbows to opposite knees cycling legs. Perform 20 reps.
208	As many rounds as possible in 12 mins:		
	(1) High Knees (30 seconds)	Legs, Core, Cardio	Run in place lifting knees high, maintain pace. Perform for 30 seconds.
	(2) Side-to-Side Push-Ups (10 reps each side)	Chest, Shoulders, Core	Shift side-to-side during push-ups, engages core. Perform 10 reps each side.
	(3) Jumping Jacks (30 seconds)	Full Body, Cardio, Legs	Jump to spread legs and clap hands overhead. Perform for 30 seconds.
209	Every minute on the minute for 20 mins:		
	(1) Pull-Ups (5 reps)	Back, Biceps, Shoulders	Pull body up on bar, chin above hands. Perform 5 reps.
	(2) Plank to Push-Up (10 reps)	Core, Shoulders, Triceps	Alternate between plank and push-up positions. Perform 10 reps.
	(3) Fire Hydrant (15 reps each leg)	Glutes, Core, Hip Flexors	On hands and knees, lift leg to side, keep knee bent. Perform 15 reps each leg.
210	45 seconds work, 15 seconds rest per exercise for 4 rounds:		
	(1) High Knees	Legs, Core, Cardio	Run in place lifting knees high, maintain pace. Perform for 45 seconds.
	(2) Plank Rotation	Core, Shoulders, Obliques	Rotate body in plank, extend arm upward, switch sides. Perform for 45 seconds.
	(3) Squat Jumps	Legs, Glutes, Cardio	Perform a squat then jump explosively. Perform for 45 seconds.
	(4) Skater Squats	Legs, Glutes, Core	Balance on one leg, squat, touch opposite hand to foot. Perform for 45 seconds.
211	As many rounds as possible in 10 mins of:		
	(1) Burpees (10 reps)	Full Body, Core, Legs	Jump, squat down, kick back into a push-up, return up. Perform 10 reps.
	(2) Reverse Plank (30 seconds)	Core, Shoulders, Back	Sit, lift body with arms, legs straight, face up. Hold for 30 seconds.
	(3) Step-Ups (15 reps each leg)	Legs, Glutes, Core	Step onto a raised platform, alternate legs. Perform 15 reps each leg.

Workout No.	Workout	Main Muscle Groups	Instructions
212	30 seconds work, 30 seconds rest per exercise for 6 rounds:		
	(1) High Knees	Legs, Core, Cardio	Run in place lifting knees high, maintain pace. Perform for 45 seconds.
	(2) Bicycle Crunches	Core, Obliques, Hip Flexors	Lie down, alternate elbows to opposite knees cycling legs. Perform for 45 seconds.
	(3) Jumping Jacks	Full Body, Cardio, Legs	Jump to spread legs and clap hands overhead. Perform for 45 seconds.
	(4) Bear Crawl	Full Body, Core, Shoulders	Crawl forward on all fours, hips down, move quickly. Perform for 45 seconds.
213	Every minute on the minute for 20 mins:		
	(1) Pull-Ups (5 reps)	Back, Biceps, Shoulders	Pull body up on bar, chin above hands. Perform 5 reps.
	(2) V-Ups (10 reps)	Core, Hip Flexors, Lower Abs	Lie back, lift legs and torso simultaneously, form 'V'. Perform 10 reps.
	(3) Glute Bridge (15 reps)	Glutes, Core, Hamstrings	Lift hips while lying on back, feet flat on ground. Perform 15 reps.
214	As many rounds as possible in 12 mins:		
	(1) Tuck Jumps (10 reps)	Legs, Core, Cardio	Jump high, tuck knees to chest mid-air. Perform 10 reps.
	(2) Side Plank (30 seconds each side)	Core, Shoulders, Obliques	Support body on one arm, side facing ground. Hold for 30 seconds each side.
	(3) Mountain Climbers (20 reps)	Core, Legs, Shoulders	Run in place in plank position, drive knees to chest. Perform 20 reps.
215	5 Rounds for time:		
	(1) Inchworm (10 reps)	Full Body, Core, Shoulders	Walk hands forward from standing, hold plank, walk back. Perform 10 reps.
	(2) Single Leg Dead Lift (10 reps each leg)	Hamstrings, Glutes, Core	Balance on one leg, hinge forward, extend free leg back. Perform 10 reps each leg.
	(3) Cross-Body Mountain Climbers (15 reps each side)	Core, Shoulders, Cardio	Bring knee towards opposite elbow while in plank position. Perform 15 reps each side.
216	45 seconds work, 15 seconds rest per exercise for 4 rounds:		
	(1) Jumping Jacks	Full Body, Cardio, Legs	Jump to spread legs and clap hands overhead. Perform for 45 seconds.
	(2) Crab Walk	Triceps, Core, Glutes	Walk backward on hands and feet, hips elevated. Perform for 45 seconds.
	(3) Flutter Kicks	Core, Hip Flexors, Lower Abs	Lie on back, alternately kick legs in small, rapid motion. Perform for 45 seconds.
	(4) Bird Dog	Core, Glutes, Shoulders	Extend opposite arm and leg, kneeling position. Perform for 45 seconds.
217	As many rounds as possible in 10 mins of:		
	(1) Squat Jumps (15 reps)	Legs, Glutes, Core	Perform a squat then jump explosively. Perform 15 reps.
	(2) Pike Push-Ups (10 reps)	Shoulders, Triceps, Core	Push-up with hips high, resembles downward dog pose. Perform 10 reps.
	(3) Reverse Crunches (20 reps)	Core, Hip Flexors, Lower Abs	Lift hips off floor, knees towards chest. Perform 20 reps.

Workout No.	Workout	Main Muscle Groups	Instructions
218	**As many rounds as possible in 12 mins:**		
	(1) High Knees (30 seconds)	Legs, Core, Cardio	Run in place lifting knees high, maintain pace. Perform for 30 seconds.
	(2) Side-to-Side Push-Ups (10 reps each side)	Chest, Shoulders, Core	Shift side-to-side during push-ups, engages core. Perform 10 reps each side.
	(3) Jumping Jacks (30 seconds)	Full Body, Cardio, Legs	Jump to spread legs and clap hands overhead. Perform for 30 seconds.
219	**Every minute on the minute for 20 mins:**		
	(1) Pull-Ups (5 reps)	Back, Biceps, Shoulders	Pull body up on bar, chin above hands. Perform 5 reps.
	(2) Plank to Push-Up (10 reps)	Core, Shoulders, Triceps	Alternate between plank and push-up positions. Perform 10 reps.
	(3) Fire Hydrant (15 reps each leg)	Glutes, Core, Hip Flexors	On hands and knees, lift leg to side, keep knee bent. Perform 15 reps each leg.
220	**45 seconds work, 15 seconds rest per exercise for 4 rounds:**		
	(1) High Knees	Legs, Core, Cardio	Run in place lifting knees high, maintain pace. Perform for 45 seconds.
	(2) Plank Rotation	Core, Shoulders, Obliques	Rotate body in plank, extend arm upward, switch sides. Perform for 45 seconds.
	(3) Squat Jumps	Legs, Glutes, Cardio	Perform a squat then jump explosively. Perform for 45 seconds.
	(4) Skater Squats	Legs, Glutes, Core	Balance on one leg, squat, touch opposite hand to foot. Perform for 45 seconds.
221	**As many rounds as possible in 10 mins of:**		
	(1) Burpees (10 reps)	Full Body, Core, Legs	Jump, squat down, kick back into a push-up, return up. Perform 10 reps.
	(2) Russian Twists (20 reps)	Core, Obliques, Hip Flexors	Twist torso holding weight, seated on ground. Perform 20 reps.
	(3) Lunge (15 reps each leg)	Legs, Glutes, Core	Step forward, lower hips to drop knee to ground. Perform 15 reps each leg.
222	**45 seconds work, 15 seconds rest per exercise for 5 rounds:**		
	(1) High Knees	Legs, Core, Cardio	Run in place lifting knees high, maintain pace. Perform for 45 seconds.
	(2) Plank with Shoulder Tap	Core, Shoulders, Triceps	In plank position, tap opposite shoulder with each hand. Perform for 45 seconds.
	(3) Jumping Jacks	Full Body, Cardio, Legs	Jump to spread legs and clap hands overhead. Perform for 45 seconds.
	(4) Flutter Kicks	Core, Hip Flexors, Lower Abs	Lie on back, alternately kick legs in small, rapid motion. Perform for 45 seconds.
223	**Every minute on the minute for 20 mins:**		
	(1) Pull-Ups (5 reps)	Back, Biceps, Shoulders	Pull body up on bar, chin above hands. Perform 5 reps.
	(2) V-Ups (10 reps)	Core, Hip Flexors, Lower Abs	Lie back, lift legs and torso simultaneously, form 'V'. Perform 10 reps.
	(3) Fire Hydrant (15 reps each leg)	Glutes, Core, Hip Flexors	On hands and knees, lift leg to side, keep knee bent. Perform 15 reps each leg.

Workout No.	Workout		Main Muscle Groups	Instructions
224	As many rounds as possible in 12 mins:			
	(1)	Tuck Jumps (10 reps)	Legs, Core, Cardio	Jump high, tuck knees to chest mid-air. Perform 10 reps.
	(2)	Side Plank (30 seconds each side)	Core, Shoulders, Obliques	Support body on one arm, side facing ground. Hold for 30 seconds each side.
	(3)	Mountain Climbers (20 reps)	Core, Legs, Shoulders	Run in place in plank position, drive knees to chest. Perform 20 reps.
225	5 Rounds for time:			
	(1)	Inchworm (10 reps)	Full Body, Core, Shoulders	Walk hands forward from standing, hold plank, walk back. Perform 10 reps.
	(2)	Single Leg Dead Lift (10 reps each leg)	Hamstrings, Glutes, Core	Balance on one leg, hinge forward, extend free leg back. Perform 10 reps each leg.
	(3)	Cross-Body Mountain Climbers (15 reps each side)	Core, Shoulders, Cardio	Bring knee towards opposite elbow while in plank position. Perform 15 reps each side.
226	45 seconds work, 15 seconds rest per exercise for 4 rounds:			
	(1)	Jumping Jacks	Full Body, Cardio, Legs	Jump to spread legs and clap hands overhead. Perform for 45 seconds.
	(2)	Crab Walk	Triceps, Core, Glutes	Walk backward on hands and feet, hips elevated. Perform for 45 seconds.
	(3)	Side Plank (each side)	Core, Obliques, Shoulders	Support body on one arm, side facing ground. Hold for 45 seconds each side.
	(4)	High Knees	Legs, Core, Cardio	Run in place lifting knees high, maintain pace. Perform for 45 seconds.
227	As many rounds as possible in 10 mins of:			
	(1)	Plank to Push-Up (10 reps)	Core, Shoulders, Triceps	Alternate between plank and push-up positions. Perform 10 reps.
	(2)	Box Jumps (15 reps)	Legs, Glutes, Core	Jump onto and off a box repeatedly, land softly. Perform 15 reps.
	(3)	Bicycle Crunches (20 reps)	Core, Obliques, Hip Flexors	Lie down, alternate elbows to opposite knees cycling legs. Perform 20 reps.
228	As many rounds as possible in 12 mins:			
	(1)	High Knees (30 seconds)	Legs, Core, Cardio	Run in place lifting knees high, maintain pace. Perform for 30 seconds.
	(2)	Side-to-Side Push-Ups (10 reps each side)	Chest, Shoulders, Core	Shift side-to-side during push-ups, engages core. Perform 10 reps each side.
	(3)	Jumping Jacks (30 seconds)	Full Body, Cardio, Legs	Jump to spread legs and clap hands overhead. Perform for 30 seconds.
229	Every minute on the minute for 20 mins:			
	(1)	Pull-Ups (5 reps)	Back, Biceps, Shoulders	Pull body up on bar, chin above hands. Perform 5 reps.
	(2)	Glute Bridge (15 reps)	Glutes, Core, Hamstrings	Lift hips while lying on back, feet flat on ground. Perform 15 reps.
	(3)	Side Lunges (10 reps each side)	Legs, Glutes, Core	Step to side into lunge, keep other leg straight. Perform 10 reps each side.

Workout No.	Workout	Main Muscle Groups	Instructions
230	**45 seconds work, 15 seconds rest per exercise for 5 rounds:**		
	(1) High Knees	Legs, Core, Cardio	Run in place lifting knees high, maintain pace. Perform for 45 seconds.
	(2) Plank with Shoulder Tap	Core, Shoulders, Triceps	In plank position, tap opposite shoulder with each hand. Perform for 45 seconds.
	(3) Squat Jumps	Legs, Glutes, Cardio	Perform a squat then jump explosively. Perform for 45 seconds.
	(4) Skater Squats	Legs, Glutes, Core	Balance on one leg, squat, touch opposite hand to foot. Perform for 45 seconds.
231	**As many rounds as possible in 10 mins of:**		
	(1) Burpees (10 reps)	Full Body, Core, Legs	Jump, squat down, kick back into a push-up, return up. Perform 10 reps.
	(2) Cross-Body Crunch (20 reps)	Core, Obliques, Hip Flexors	Touch opposite knee to elbow, lying down. Perform 20 reps.
	(3) Walking Lunges (15 reps each leg)	Legs, Glutes, Core	Step forward into a lunge, move forward alternating legs. Perform 15 reps each leg.
232	**45 seconds work, 15 seconds rest per exercise for 4 rounds:**		
	(1) High Knees	Legs, Core, Cardio	Run in place lifting knees high, maintain pace. Perform for 45 seconds.
	(2) Side-to-Side Push-Ups	Chest, Shoulders, Core	Shift side-to-side during push-ups, engages core. Perform for 45 seconds.
	(3) Jumping Jacks	Full Body, Cardio, Legs	Jump to spread legs and clap hands overhead. Perform for 45 seconds.
	(4) Flutter Kicks	Core, Hip Flexors, Lower Abs	Lie on back, alternately kick legs in small, rapid motion. Perform for 45 seconds.
233	**Every minute on the minute for 20 mins:**		
	(1) Pull-Ups (5 reps)	Back, Biceps, Shoulders	Pull body up on bar, chin above hands. Perform 5 reps.
	(2) Plank with Shoulder Tap (10 reps each side)	Core, Shoulders, Triceps	In plank position, tap opposite shoulder with each hand. Perform 10 reps each side.
	(3) Single Leg Squat (10 reps each leg)	Legs, Glutes, Core	Stand on one leg, squat, maintain balance. Perform 10 reps each leg.
234	**As many rounds as possible in 12 mins:**		
	(1) Tuck Jumps (10 reps)	Legs, Core, Cardio	Jump high, tuck knees to chest mid-air. Perform 10 reps.
	(2) Bird Dog (10 reps each side)	Core, Glutes, Shoulders	Extend opposite arm and leg, kneeling position. Perform 10 reps each side.
	(3) Mountain Climbers (20 reps)	Core, Legs, Shoulders	Run in place in plank position, drive knees to chest. Perform 20 reps.
235	**5 Rounds for time:**		
	(1) Inchworm (10 reps)	Full Body, Core, Shoulders	Walk hands forward from standing, hold plank, walk back. Perform 10 reps.
	(2) Side Lunges (10 reps each side)	Legs, Glutes, Core	Step to side into lunge, keep other leg straight. Perform 10 reps each side.
	(3) Cross-Body Mountain Climbers (15 reps each side)	Core, Shoulders, Cardio	Bring knee towards opposite elbow while in plank position. Perform 15 reps each side.

Workout No.	Workout	Main Muscle Groups	Instructions
236	45 seconds work, 15 seconds rest per exercise for 5 rounds:		
	(1) Jumping Jacks	Full Body, Cardio, Legs	Jump to spread legs and clap hands overhead. Perform for 45 seconds.
	(2) Crab Walk	Triceps, Core, Glutes	Walk backward on hands and feet, hips elevated. Perform for 45 seconds.
	(3) Scissor Kick	Core, Hip Flexors, Lower Abs	Alternately lift legs in lying position, engages core. Perform for 45 seconds.
	(4) High Knees	Legs, Core, Cardio	Run in place lifting knees high, maintain pace. Perform for 45 seconds.
237	As many rounds as possible in 10 mins of:		
	(1) Burpee to Pull-Up (10 reps)	Full Body, Core, Back	Perform a burpee, then a pull-up. Perform 10 reps.
	(2) Lying Leg Lift (15 reps)	Core, Hip Flexors, Lower Abs	Raise legs vertically, lying flat on back. Perform 15 reps.
	(3) Glute Bridge (20 reps)	Glutes, Core, Hamstrings	Lift hips while lying on back, feet flat on ground. Perform 20 reps.
238	As many rounds as possible in 12 mins:		
	(1) High Knees (30 seconds)	Legs, Core, Cardio	Run in place lifting knees high, maintain pace. Perform for 30 seconds.
	(2) Wide/Narrow Push-Ups (10 reps)	Chest, Shoulders, Triceps	Perform push-ups with varying hand widths. Perform 10 reps.
	(3) Jumping Jacks (30 seconds)	Full Body, Cardio, Legs	Jump to spread legs and clap hands overhead. Perform for 30 seconds.
239	Every minute on the minute for 20 mins:		
	(1) Pull-Ups (5 reps)	Back, Biceps, Shoulders	Pull body up on bar, chin above hands. Perform 5 reps.
	(2) V-Ups (10 reps)	Core, Hip Flexors, Lower Abs	Lie back, lift legs and torso simultaneously, form 'V'. Perform 10 reps.
	(3) Donkey Kicks (15 reps each leg)	Glutes, Core, Hamstrings	On hands and knees, kick one leg back and up. Perform 15 reps each leg.
240	50 seconds work, 10 seconds rest per exercise for 5 rounds:		
	(1) High Knees	Legs, Core, Cardio	Run in place lifting knees high, maintain pace. Perform for 45 seconds.
	(2) Plank with Shoulder Tap	Core, Shoulders, Triceps	In plank position, tap opposite shoulder with each hand. Perform for 45 seconds.
	(3) Squat Jumps	Legs, Glutes, Cardio	Perform a squat then jump explosively. Perform for 45 seconds.
	(4) Bird Dog	Core, Glutes, Shoulders	Extend opposite arm and leg, kneeling position. Perform for 45 seconds.
241	As many rounds as possible in 10 mins of:		
	(1) Burpees (10 reps)	Full Body, Core, Legs	Jump, squat down, kick back into a push-up, return up. Perform 10 reps.
	(2) Russian Twists (20 reps)	Core, Obliques, Hip Flexors	Twist torso holding weight, seated on ground. Perform 20 reps.
	(3) Step-Ups (15 reps each leg)	Legs, Glutes, Core	Step onto a raised platform, alternate legs. Perform 15 reps each leg.

Workout No.	Workout		Main Muscle Groups	Instructions
242	45 seconds work, 15 seconds rest per exercise for 4 rounds:			
	(1)	High Knees	Legs, Core, Cardio	Run in place lifting knees high, maintain pace. Perform for 45 seconds.
	(2)	Bicycle Crunches	Core, Obliques, Hip Flexors	Lie down, alternate elbows to opposite knees cycling legs. Perform for 45 seconds.
	(3)	Jumping Jacks	Full Body, Cardio, Legs	Jump to spread legs and clap hands overhead. Perform for 45 seconds.
	(4)	Bear Crawl	Full Body, Core, Shoulders	Crawl forward on all fours, hips down, move quickly. Perform for 45 seconds.
243	Every minute on the minute for 20 mins:			
	(1)	Pull-Ups (5 reps)	Back, Biceps, Shoulders	Pull body up on bar, chin above hands. Perform 5 reps.
	(2)	V-Ups (10 reps)	Core, Hip Flexors, Lower Abs	Lie back, lift legs and torso simultaneously, form 'V'. Perform 10 reps.
	(3)	Fire Hydrant (15 reps each leg)	Glutes, Core, Hip Flexors	On hands and knees, lift leg to side, keep knee bent. Perform 15 reps each leg.
244	As many rounds as possible in 12 mins:			
	(1)	Tuck Jumps (10 reps)	Legs, Core, Cardio	Jump high, tuck knees to chest mid-air. Perform 10 reps.
	(2)	Side Plank (30 seconds each side)	Core, Shoulders, Obliques	Support body on one arm, side facing ground. Hold for 30 seconds each side.
	(3)	Mountain Climbers (20 reps)	Core, Legs, Shoulders	Run in place in plank position, drive knees to chest. Perform 20 reps.
245	5 Rounds for time:			
	(1)	Inchworm (10 reps)	Full Body, Core, Shoulders	Walk hands forward from standing, hold plank, walk back. Perform 10 reps.
	(2)	Single Leg Dead Lift (10 reps each leg)	Hamstrings, Glutes, Core	Balance on one leg, hinge forward, extend free leg back. Perform 10 reps each leg.
	(3)	Cross-Body Mountain Climbers (15 reps each side)	Core, Shoulders, Cardio	Bring knee towards opposite elbow while in plank position. Perform 15 reps each side.
246	45 seconds work, 15 seconds rest per exercise for 5 rounds:			
	(1)	Jumping Jacks	Full Body, Cardio, Legs	Jump to spread legs and clap hands overhead. Perform for 45 seconds.
	(2)	Crab Walk	Triceps, Core, Glutes	Walk backward on hands and feet, hips elevated. Perform for 45 seconds.
	(3)	Flutter Kicks	Core, Hip Flexors, Lower Abs	Lie on back, alternately kick legs in small, rapid motion. Perform for 45 seconds.
	(4)	Bird Dog	Core, Glutes, Shoulders	Extend opposite arm and leg, kneeling position. Perform for 45 seconds.
247	As many rounds as possible in 10 mins of:			
	(1)	Squat Jumps (15 reps)	Legs, Glutes, Core	Perform a squat then jump explosively. Perform 15 reps.
	(2)	Pike Push-Ups (10 reps)	Shoulders, Triceps, Core	Push-up with hips high, resembles downward dog pose. Perform 10 reps.
	(3)	Reverse Crunches (20 reps)	Core, Hip Flexors, Lower Abs	Lift hips off floor, knees towards chest. Perform 20 reps.

Workout No.	Workout	Main Muscle Groups	Instructions
248	As many rounds as possible in 12 mins:		
	(1) High Knees (30 seconds)	Legs, Core, Cardio	Run in place lifting knees high, maintain pace. Perform for 30 seconds.
	(2) Side-to-Side Push-Ups (10 reps each side)	Chest, Shoulders, Core	Shift side-to-side during push-ups, engages core. Perform 10 reps each side.
	(3) Jumping Jacks (30 seconds)	Full Body, Cardio, Legs	Jump to spread legs and clap hands overhead. Perform for 30 seconds.
249	Every minute on the minute for 20 mins:		
	(1) Pull-Ups (5 reps)	Back, Biceps, Shoulders	Pull body up on bar, chin above hands. Perform 5 reps.
	(2) Plank to Push-Up (10 reps)	Core, Shoulders, Triceps	Alternate between plank and push-up positions. Perform 10 reps.
	(3) Fire Hydrant (15 reps each leg)	Glutes, Core, Hip Flexors	On hands and knees, lift leg to side, keep knee bent. Perform 15 reps each leg.
250	45 seconds work, 15 seconds rest per exercise for 4 rounds:		
	(1) High Knees	Legs, Core, Cardio	Run in place lifting knees high, maintain pace. Perform for 45 seconds.
	(2) Plank Rotation	Core, Shoulders, Obliques	Rotate body in plank, extend arm upward, switch sides. Perform for 45 seconds.
	(3) Squat Jumps	Legs, Glutes, Cardio	Perform a squat then jump explosively. Perform for 45 seconds.
	(4) Skater Squats	Legs, Glutes, Core	Balance on one leg, squat, touch opposite hand to foot. Perform for 45 seconds.
251	As many rounds as possible in 10 mins of:		
	(1) Burpees (10 reps)	Full Body, Core, Legs	Jump, squat down, kick back into a push-up, return up. Perform 10 reps.
	(2) Side Plank (30 seconds each side)	Core, Shoulders, Obliques	Support body on one arm, side facing ground. Hold for 30 seconds each side.
	(3) Step-Ups (15 reps each leg)	Legs, Glutes, Core	Step onto a raised platform, alternate legs. Perform 15 reps each leg.
252	45 seconds work, 15 seconds rest per exercise for 4 rounds:		
	(1) High Knees	Legs, Core, Cardio	Run in place lifting knees high, maintain pace. Perform for 45 seconds.
	(2) Cross-Body Mountain Climbers	Core, Obliques, Shoulders	Bring knee towards opposite elbow while in plank position. Perform for 45 seconds.
	(3) Jumping Jacks	Full Body, Cardio, Legs	Jump to spread legs and clap hands overhead. Perform for 45 seconds.
	(4) Bird Dog	Core, Glutes, Shoulders	Extend opposite arm and leg, kneeling position. Perform for 45 seconds.
253	Every minute on the minute for 20 mins:		
	(1) Pull-Ups (5 reps)	Back, Biceps, Shoulders	Pull body up on bar, chin above hands. Perform 5 reps.
	(2) V-Ups (10 reps)	Core, Hip Flexors, Lower Abs	Lie back, lift legs and torso simultaneously, form 'V'. Perform 10 reps.
	(3) Glute Bridge (15 reps)	Glutes, Core, Hamstrings	Lift hips while lying on back, feet flat on ground. Perform 15 reps.

Workout No.	Workout		Main Muscle Groups	Instructions
254	As many rounds as possible in 12 mins:			
	(1)	Tuck Jumps (10 reps)	Legs, Core, Cardio	Jump high, tuck knees to chest mid-air. Perform 10 reps.
	(2)	Dolphin Kicks (15 reps)	Core, Hip Flexors, Legs	Lie face down, kick legs like a dolphin's tail. Perform 15 reps.
	(3)	Mountain Climbers (20 reps)	Core, Legs, Shoulders	Run in place in plank position, drive knees to chest. Perform 20 reps.
255	5 Rounds for time:			
	(1)	Inchworm (10 reps)	Full Body, Core, Shoulders	Walk hands forward from standing, hold plank, walk back. Perform 10 reps.
	(2)	Single Leg Dead Lift (10 reps each leg)	Hamstrings, Glutes, Core	Balance on one leg, hinge forward, extend free leg back. Perform 10 reps each leg.
	(3)	Side Lunges (15 reps each side)	Legs, Glutes, Core	Step to side into lunge, keep other leg straight. Perform 15 reps each side.
256	45 seconds work, 15 seconds rest per exercise for 4 rounds:			
	(1)	Jumping Jacks	Full Body, Cardio, Legs	Jump to spread legs and clap hands overhead. Perform for 45 seconds.
	(2)	Crab Walk	Triceps, Core, Glutes	Walk backward on hands and feet, hips elevated. Perform for 45 seconds.
	(3)	Flutter Kicks	Core, Hip Flexors, Lower Abs	Lie on back, alternately kick legs in small, rapid motion. Perform for 45 seconds.
	(4)	Skater Squats	Legs, Glutes, Core	Balance on one leg, squat, touch opposite hand to foot. Perform for 45 seconds.
257	As many rounds as possible in 10 mins of:			
	(1)	Squat Jumps (15 reps)	Legs, Glutes, Core	Perform a squat then jump explosively. Perform 15 reps.
	(2)	Pike Push-Ups (10 reps)	Shoulders, Triceps, Core	Push-up with hips high, resembles downward dog pose. Perform 10 reps.
	(3)	Bicycle Crunches (20 reps)	Core, Obliques, Hip Flexors	Lie down, alternate elbows to opposite knees cycling legs. Perform 20 reps.
258	As many rounds as possible in 12 mins:			
	(1)	High Knees (30 seconds)	Legs, Core, Cardio	Run in place lifting knees high, maintain pace. Perform for 30 seconds.
	(2)	Side-to-Side Push-Ups (10 reps each side)	Chest, Shoulders, Core	Shift side-to-side during push-ups, engages core. Perform 10 reps each side.
	(3)	Jumping Jacks (30 seconds)	Full Body, Cardio, Legs	Jump to spread legs and clap hands overhead. Perform for 30 seconds.
259	Every minute on the minute for 20 mins:			
	(1)	Pull-Ups (5 reps)	Back, Biceps, Shoulders	Pull body up on bar, chin above hands. Perform 5 reps.
	(2)	Plank to Push-Up (10 reps)	Core, Shoulders, Triceps	Alternate between plank and push-up positions. Perform 10 reps.
	(3)	Fire Hydrant (15 reps each leg)	Glutes, Core, Hip Flexors	On hands and knees, lift leg to side, keep knee bent. Perform 15 reps each leg.

Workout No.	Workout	Main Muscle Groups	Instructions
260	**40 seconds work, 20 seconds rest per exercise for 8 rounds:**		
	(1) High Knees	Legs, Core, Cardio	Run in place lifting knees high, maintain pace. Perform for 45 seconds.
	(2) Plank Rotation	Core, Shoulders, Obliques	Rotate body in plank, extend arm upward, switch sides. Perform for 45 seconds.
	(3) Squat Jumps	Legs, Glutes, Cardio	Perform a squat then jump explosively. Perform for 45 seconds.
	(4) Bird Dog	Core, Glutes, Shoulders	Extend opposite arm and leg, kneeling position. Perform for 45 seconds.
261	**As many rounds as possible in 10 mins of:**		
	(1) Burpees (10 reps)	Full Body, Core, Legs	Jump, squat down, kick back into a push-up, return up. Perform 10 reps.
	(2) Russian Twists (20 reps)	Core, Obliques, Hip Flexors	Twist torso holding weight, seated on ground. Perform 20 reps.
	(3) Walking Lunges (15 reps each leg)	Legs, Glutes, Core	Step forward into a lunge, move forward alternating legs. Perform 15 reps each leg.
262	**45 seconds work, 15 seconds rest per exercise for 4 rounds:**		
	(1) High Knees	Legs, Core, Cardio	Run in place lifting knees high, maintain pace. Perform for 45 seconds.
	(2) Side-to-Side Push-Ups	Chest, Shoulders, Core	Shift side-to-side during push-ups, engages core. Perform for 45 seconds.
	(3) Jumping Jacks	Full Body, Cardio, Legs	Jump to spread legs and clap hands overhead. Perform for 45 seconds.
	(4) Flutter Kicks	Core, Hip Flexors, Lower Abs	Lie on back, alternately kick legs in small, rapid motion. Perform for 45 seconds.
263	**Every minute on the minute for 20 mins:**		
	(1) Pull-Ups (5 reps)	Back, Biceps, Shoulders	Pull body up on bar, chin above hands. Perform 5 reps.
	(2) Plank with Shoulder Tap (10 reps each side)	Core, Shoulders, Triceps	In plank position, tap opposite shoulder with each hand. Perform 10 reps each side.
	(3) Single Leg Squat (10 reps each leg)	Legs, Glutes, Core	Stand on one leg, squat, maintain balance. Perform 10 reps each leg.
264	**As many rounds as possible in 12 mins:**		
	(1) Tuck Jumps (10 reps)	Legs, Core, Cardio	Jump high, tuck knees to chest mid-air. Perform 10 reps.
	(2) Bird Dog (10 reps each side)	Core, Glutes, Shoulders	Extend opposite arm and leg, kneeling position. Perform 10 reps each side.
	(3) Mountain Climbers (20 reps)	Core, Legs, Shoulders	Run in place in plank position, drive knees to chest. Perform 20 reps.
265	**5 Rounds for time:**		
	(1) Inchworm (10 reps)	Full Body, Core, Shoulders	Walk hands forward from standing, hold plank, walk back. Perform 10 reps.
	(2) Side Lunges (10 reps each side)	Legs, Glutes, Core	Step to side into lunge, keep other leg straight. Perform 10 reps each side.
	(3) Cross-Body Mountain Climbers (15 reps each side)	Core, Shoulders, Cardio	Bring knee towards opposite elbow while in plank position. Perform 15 reps each side.

Workout No.	Workout		Main Muscle Groups	Instructions
266	45 seconds work, 15 seconds rest per exercise for 4 rounds:			
	(1)	Jumping Jacks	Full Body, Cardio, Legs	Jump to spread legs and clap hands overhead. Perform for 45 seconds.
	(2)	Crab Walk	Triceps, Core, Glutes	Walk backward on hands and feet, hips elevated. Perform for 45 seconds.
	(3)	Scissor Kicks	Core, Hip Flexors, Lower Abs	Alternately lift legs in lying position, engages core. Perform for 45 seconds.
	(4)	High Knees	Legs, Core, Cardio	Run in place lifting knees high, maintain pace. Perform for 45 seconds.
267	As many rounds as possible in 10 mins of:			
	(1)	Burpee to Pull-Up (10 reps)	Full Body, Core, Back	Perform a burpee, then a pull-up. Perform 10 reps.
	(2)	Lying Leg Lift (15 reps)	Core, Hip Flexors, Lower Abs	Raise legs vertically, lying flat on back. Perform 15 reps.
	(3)	Glute Bridge (20 reps)	Glutes, Core, Hamstrings	Lift hips while lying on back, feet flat on ground. Perform 20 reps.
268	As many rounds as possible in 12 mins:			
	(1)	High Knees (30 seconds)	Legs, Core, Cardio	Run in place lifting knees high, maintain pace. Perform for 30 seconds.
	(2)	Wide/Narrow Push-Ups (10 reps)	Chest, Shoulders, Triceps	Perform push-ups with varying hand widths. Perform 10 reps.
	(3)	Jumping Jacks (30 seconds)	Full Body, Cardio, Legs	Jump to spread legs and clap hands overhead. Perform for 30 seconds.
269	Every minute on the minute for 20 mins:			
	(1)	Pull-Ups (5 reps)	Back, Biceps, Shoulders	Pull body up on bar, chin above hands. Perform 5 reps.
	(2)	V-Ups (10 reps)	Core, Hip Flexors, Lower Abs	Lie back, lift legs and torso simultaneously, form 'V'. Perform 10 reps.
	(3)	Donkey Kicks (15 reps each leg)	Glutes, Core, Hamstrings	On hands and knees, kick one leg back and up. Perform 15 reps each leg.
270	45 seconds work, 15 seconds rest per exercise for 4 rounds:			
	(1)	High Knees	Legs, Core, Cardio	Run in place lifting knees high, maintain pace. Perform for 45 seconds.
	(2)	Plank with Shoulder Tap	Core, Shoulders, Triceps	In plank position, tap opposite shoulder with each hand. Perform for 45 seconds.
	(3)	Squat Jumps	Legs, Glutes, Cardio	Perform a squat then jump explosively. Perform for 45 seconds.
	(4)	Bird Dog	Core, Glutes, Shoulders	Extend opposite arm and leg, kneeling position. Perform for 45 seconds.
271	As many rounds as possible in 10 mins of:			
	(1)	Burpees (10 reps)	Full Body, Core, Legs	Jump, squat down, kick back into a push-up, return up. Perform 10 reps.
	(2)	Russian Twists (20 reps)	Core, Obliques, Hip Flexors	Twist torso holding weight, seated on ground. Perform 20 reps.
	(3)	Lunge (15 reps each leg)	Legs, Glutes, Core	Step forward, lower hips to drop knee to ground. Perform 15 reps each leg.

Workout No.	Workout	Main Muscle Groups	Instructions
272	**30 seconds work, 30 seconds rest per exercise for 9 rounds:**		
(1)	High Knees	Legs, Core, Cardio	Run in place lifting knees high, maintain pace. Perform for 45 seconds.
(2)	Side-to-Side Push-Ups	Chest, Shoulders, Core	Shift side-to-side during push-ups, engages core. Perform for 45 seconds.
(3)	Jumping Jacks	Full Body, Cardio, Legs	Jump to spread legs and clap hands overhead. Perform for 45 seconds.
(4)	Flutter Kicks	Core, Hip Flexors, Lower Abs	Lie on back, alternately kick legs in small, rapid motion. Perform for 45 seconds.
273	**Every minute on the minute for 20 mins:**		
(1)	Pull-Ups (5 reps)	Back, Biceps, Shoulders	Pull body up on bar, chin above hands. Perform 5 reps.
(2)	Plank with Shoulder Tap (10 reps each side)	Core, Shoulders, Triceps	In plank position, tap opposite shoulder with each hand. Perform 10 reps each side.
(3)	Single Leg Squat (10 reps each leg)	Legs, Glutes, Core	Stand on one leg, squat, maintain balance. Perform 10 reps each leg.
274	**As many rounds as possible in 12 mins:**		
(1)	Tuck Jumps (10 reps)	Legs, Core, Cardio	Jump high, tuck knees to chest mid-air. Perform 10 reps.
(2)	Bird Dog (10 reps each side)	Core, Glutes, Shoulders	Extend opposite arm and leg, kneeling position. Perform 10 reps each side.
(3)	Mountain Climbers (20 reps)	Core, Legs, Shoulders	Run in place in plank position, drive knees to chest. Perform 20 reps.
275	**5 Rounds for time:**		
(1)	Inchworm (10 reps)	Full Body, Core, Shoulders	Walk hands forward from standing, hold plank, walk back. Perform 10 reps.
(2)	Side Lunges (10 reps each side)	Legs, Glutes, Core	Step to side into lunge, keep other leg straight. Perform 10 reps each side.
(3)	Cross-Body Mountain Climbers (15 reps each side)	Core, Shoulders, Cardio	Bring knee towards opposite elbow while in plank position. Perform 15 reps each side.
276	**45 seconds work, 15 seconds rest per exercise for 4 rounds:**		
(1)	Jumping Jacks	Full Body, Cardio, Legs	Jump to spread legs and clap hands overhead. Perform for 45 seconds.
(2)	Crab Walk	Triceps, Core, Glutes	Walk backward on hands and feet, hips elevated. Perform for 45 seconds.
(3)	Scissor Kicks	Core, Hip Flexors, Lower Abs	Alternately lift legs in lying position, engages core. Perform for 45 seconds.
(4)	High Knees	Legs, Core, Cardio	Run in place lifting knees high, maintain pace. Perform for 45 seconds.
277	**As many rounds as possible in 10 mins of:**		
(1)	Burpee to Pull-Up (10 reps)	Full Body, Core, Back	Perform a burpee, then a pull-up. Perform 10 reps.
(2)	Lying Leg Lift (15 reps)	Core, Hip Flexors, Lower Abs	Raise legs vertically, lying flat on back. Perform 15 reps.
(3)	Glute Bridge (20 reps)	Glutes, Core, Hamstrings	Lift hips while lying on back, feet flat on ground. Perform 20 reps.

Workout No.	Workout	Main Muscle Groups	Instructions
278	As many rounds as possible in 12 mins:		
(1)	High Knees (30 seconds)	Legs, Core, Cardio	Run in place lifting knees high, maintain pace. Perform for 30 seconds.
(2)	Wide/Narrow Push-Ups (10 reps)	Chest, Shoulders, Triceps	Perform push-ups with varying hand widths. Perform 10 reps.
(3)	Jumping Jacks (30 seconds)	Full Body, Cardio, Legs	Jump to spread legs and clap hands overhead. Perform for 30 seconds.
279	Every minute on the minute for 20 mins:		
(1)	Pull-Ups (5 reps)	Back, Biceps, Shoulders	Pull body up on bar, chin above hands. Perform 5 reps.
(2)	V-Ups (10 reps)	Core, Hip Flexors, Lower Abs	Lie back, lift legs and torso simultaneously, form 'V'. Perform 10 reps.
(3)	Donkey Kicks (15 reps each leg)	Glutes, Core, Hamstrings	On hands and knees, kick one leg back and up. Perform 15 reps each leg.
280	45 seconds work, 15 seconds rest per exercise for 5 rounds:		
(1)	High Knees	Legs, Core, Cardio	Run in place lifting knees high, maintain pace. Perform for 45 seconds.
(2)	Plank with Shoulder Tap	Core, Shoulders, Triceps	In plank position, tap opposite shoulder with each hand. Perform for 45 seconds.
(3)	Squat Jumps	Legs, Glutes, Cardio	Perform a squat then jump explosively. Perform for 45 seconds.
(4)	Bird Dog	Core, Glutes, Shoulders	Extend opposite arm and leg, kneeling position. Perform for 45 seconds.
281	As many rounds as possible in 10 mins of:		
(1)	Burpees (10 reps)	Full Body, Core, Legs	Jump, squat down, kick back into a push-up, return up. Perform 10 reps.
(2)	Russian Twists (20 reps)	Core, Obliques, Hip Flexors	Twist torso holding weight, seated on ground. Perform 20 reps.
(3)	Lunge (15 reps each leg)	Legs, Glutes, Core	Step forward, lower hips to drop knee to ground. Perform 15 reps each leg.
282	45 seconds work, 15 seconds rest per exercise for 4 rounds:		
(1)	High Knees	Legs, Core, Cardio	Run in place lifting knees high, maintain pace. Perform for 45 seconds.
(2)	Plank Rotation	Core, Shoulders, Obliques	Rotate body in plank, extend arm upward, switch sides. Perform for 45 seconds.
(3)	Jumping Jacks	Full Body, Cardio, Legs	Jump to spread legs and clap hands overhead. Perform for 45 seconds.
(4)	Bear Crawl	Full Body, Core, Shoulders	Crawl forward on all fours, hips down, move quickly. Perform for 45 seconds.
283	Every minute on the minute for 20 mins:		
(1)	Pull-Ups (5 reps)	Back, Biceps, Shoulders	Pull body up on bar, chin above hands. Perform 5 reps.
(2)	V-Ups (10 reps)	Core, Hip Flexors, Lower Abs	Lie back, lift legs and torso simultaneously, form 'V'. Perform 10 reps.
(3)	Glute Bridge (15 reps)	Glutes, Core, Hamstrings	Lift hips while lying on back, feet flat on ground. Perform 15 reps.

Workout No.	Workout		Main Muscle Groups	Instructions
284	**As many rounds as possible in 12 mins:**			
	(1)	Tuck Jumps (10 reps)	Legs, Core, Cardio	Jump high, tuck knees to chest mid-air. Perform 10 reps.
	(2)	Bicycle Crunches (15 reps)	Core, Obliques, Hip Flexors	Lie down, alternate elbows to opposite knees cycling legs. Perform 15 reps.
	(3)	Mountain Climbers (20 reps)	Core, Legs, Shoulders	Run in place in plank position, drive knees to chest. Perform 20 reps.
285	**5 Rounds for time:**			
	(1)	Inchworm (10 reps)	Full Body, Core, Shoulders	Walk hands forward from standing, hold plank, walk back. Perform 10 reps.
	(2)	Side Lunges (10 reps each side)	Legs, Glutes, Core	Step to side into lunge, keep other leg straight. Perform 10 reps each side.
	(3)	Cross-Body Mountain Climbers (15 reps each side)	Core, Shoulders, Cardio	Bring knee towards opposite elbow while in plank position. Perform 15 reps each side.
286	**45 seconds work, 15 seconds rest per exercise for 4 rounds:**			
	(1)	Jumping Jacks	Full Body, Cardio, Legs	Jump to spread legs and clap hands overhead. Perform for 45 seconds.
	(2)	Crab Walk	Triceps, Core, Glutes	Walk backward on hands and feet, hips elevated. Perform for 45 seconds.
	(3)	Flutter Kicks	Core, Hip Flexors, Lower Abs	Lie on back, alternately kick legs in small, rapid motion. Perform for 45 seconds.
	(4)	Bird Dog	Core, Glutes, Shoulders	Extend opposite arm and leg, kneeling position. Perform for 45 seconds.
287	**As many rounds as possible in 10 mins of:**			
	(1)	Squat Jumps (15 reps)	Legs, Glutes, Core	Perform a squat then jump explosively. Perform 15 reps.
	(2)	Pike Push-Ups (10 reps)	Shoulders, Triceps, Core	Push-up with hips high, resembles downward dog pose. Perform 10 reps.
	(3)	Reverse Crunches (20 reps)	Core, Hip Flexors, Lower Abs	Lift hips off floor, knees towards chest. Perform 20 reps.
288	**As many rounds as possible in 12 mins:**			
	(1)	High Knees (30 seconds)	Legs, Core, Cardio	Run in place lifting knees high, maintain pace. Perform for 30 seconds.
	(2)	Side-to-Side Push-Ups (10 reps each side)	Chest, Shoulders, Core	Shift side-to-side during push-ups, engages core. Perform 10 reps each side.
	(3)	Jumping Jacks (30 seconds)	Full Body, Cardio, Legs	Jump to spread legs and clap hands overhead. Perform for 30 seconds.
289	**Every minute on the minute for 20 mins:**			
	(1)	Pull-Ups (5 reps)	Back, Biceps, Shoulders	Pull body up on bar, chin above hands. Perform 5 reps.
	(2)	Plank to Push-Up (10 reps)	Core, Shoulders, Triceps	Alternate between plank and push-up positions. Perform 10 reps.
	(3)	Fire Hydrant (15 reps each leg)	Glutes, Core, Hip Flexors	On hands and knees, lift leg to side, keep knee bent. Perform 15 reps each leg.

Workout No.	Workout	Main Muscle Groups	Instructions
290	**45 seconds work, 15 seconds rest per exercise for 5 rounds:**		
	(1) High Knees	Legs, Core, Cardio	Run in place lifting knees high, maintain pace. Perform for 45 seconds.
	(2) Plank Rotation	Core, Shoulders, Obliques	Rotate body in plank, extend arm upward, switch sides. Perform for 45 seconds.
	(3) Squat Jumps	Legs, Glutes, Cardio	Perform a squat then jump explosively. Perform for 45 seconds.
	(4) Skater Squats	Legs, Glutes, Core	Balance on one leg, squat, touch opposite hand to foot. Perform for 45 seconds.
291	**As many rounds as possible in 10 mins of:**		
	(1) Burpees (10 reps)	Full Body, Core, Legs	Jump, squat down, kick back into a push-up, return up. Perform 10 reps.
	(2) Russian Twists (20 reps)	Core, Obliques, Hip Flexors	Twist torso holding weight, seated on ground. Perform 20 reps.
	(3) Step-Ups (15 reps each leg)	Legs, Glutes, Core	Step onto a raised platform, alternate legs. Perform 15 reps each leg.
292	**45 seconds work, 15 seconds rest per exercise for 4 rounds:**		
	(1) High Knees	Legs, Core, Cardio	Run in place lifting knees high, maintain pace. Perform for 45 seconds.
	(2) Bicycle Crunches	Core, Obliques, Hip Flexors	Lie down, alternate elbows to opposite knees cycling legs. Perform for 45 seconds.
	(3) Jumping Jacks	Full Body, Cardio, Legs	Jump to spread legs and clap hands overhead. Perform for 45 seconds.
	(4) Bear Crawl	Full Body, Core, Shoulders	Crawl forward on all fours, hips down, move quickly. Perform for 45 seconds.
293	**Every minute on the minute for 20 mins:**		
	(1) Pull-Ups (5 reps)	Back, Biceps, Shoulders	Pull body up on bar, chin above hands. Perform 5 reps.
	(2) V-Ups (10 reps)	Core, Hip Flexors, Lower Abs	Lie back, lift legs and torso simultaneously, form 'V'. Perform 10 reps.
	(3) Fire Hydrant (15 reps each leg)	Glutes, Core, Hip Flexors	On hands and knees, lift leg to side, keep knee bent. Perform 15 reps each leg.
294	**As many rounds as possible in 12 mins:**		
	(1) Tuck Jumps (10 reps)	Legs, Core, Cardio	Jump high, tuck knees to chest mid-air. Perform 10 reps.
	(2) Side Plank (30 seconds each side)	Core, Shoulders, Obliques	Support body on one arm, side facing ground. Hold for 30 seconds each side.
	(3) Mountain Climbers (20 reps)	Core, Legs, Shoulders	Run in place in plank position, drive knees to chest. Perform 20 reps.
295	**5 Rounds for time:**		
	(1) Inchworm (10 reps)	Full Body, Core, Shoulders	Walk hands forward from standing, hold plank, walk back. Perform 10 reps.
	(2) Single Leg Dead Lift (10 reps each leg)	Hamstrings, Glutes, Core	Balance on one leg, hinge forward, extend free leg back. Perform 10 reps each leg.
	(3) Cross-Body Mountain Climbers (15 reps each side)	Core, Shoulders, Cardio	Bring knee towards opposite elbow while in plank position. Perform 15 reps each side.

Workout No.	Workout		Main Muscle Groups	Instructions
296	**45 seconds work, 15 seconds rest per exercise for 4 rounds:**			
	(1)	Jumping Jacks	Full Body, Cardio, Legs	Jump to spread legs and clap hands overhead. Perform for 45 seconds.
	(2)	Crab Walk	Triceps, Core, Glutes	Walk backward on hands and feet, hips elevated. Perform for 45 seconds.
	(3)	Flutter Kicks	Core, Hip Flexors, Lower Abs	Lie on back, alternately kick legs in small, rapid motion. Perform for 45 seconds.
	(4)	Bird Dog	Core, Glutes, Shoulders	Extend opposite arm and leg, kneeling position. Perform for 45 seconds.
297	**As many rounds as possible in 10 mins of:**			
	(1)	Squat Jumps (15 reps)	Legs, Glutes, Core	Perform a squat then jump explosively. Perform 15 reps.
	(2)	Pike Push-Ups (10 reps)	Shoulders, Triceps, Core	Push-up with hips high, resembles downward dog pose. Perform 10 reps.
	(3)	Bicycle Crunches (20 reps)	Core, Obliques, Hip Flexors	Lie down, alternate elbows to opposite knees cycling legs. Perform 20 reps.
298	**As many rounds as possible in 12 mins:**			
	(1)	High Knees (30 seconds)	Legs, Core, Cardio	Run in place lifting knees high, maintain pace. Perform for 30 seconds.
	(2)	Side-to-Side Push-Ups (10 reps each side)	Chest, Shoulders, Core	Shift side-to-side during push-ups, engages core. Perform 10 reps each side.
	(3)	Jumping Jacks (30 seconds)	Full Body, Cardio, Legs	Jump to spread legs and clap hands overhead. Perform for 30 seconds.
299	**Every minute on the minute for 20 mins:**			
	(1)	Pull-Ups (5 reps)	Back, Biceps, Shoulders	Pull body up on bar, chin above hands. Perform 5 reps.
	(2)	Plank to Push-Up (10 reps)	Core, Shoulders, Triceps	Alternate between plank and push-up positions. Perform 10 reps.
	(3)	Donkey Kicks (15 reps each leg)	Glutes, Core, Hamstrings	On hands and knees, kick one leg back and up. Perform 15 reps each leg.
300	**45 seconds work, 15 seconds rest per exercise for 4 rounds:**			
	(1)	High Knees	Legs, Core, Cardio	Run in place lifting knees high, maintain pace. Perform for 45 seconds.
	(2)	Plank Rotation	Core, Shoulders, Obliques	Rotate body in plank, extend arm upward, switch sides. Perform for 45 seconds.
	(3)	Squat Jumps	Legs, Glutes, Cardio	Perform a squat then jump explosively. Perform for 45 seconds.
	(4)	Skater Squats	Legs, Glutes, Core	Balance on one leg, squat, touch opposite hand to foot. Perform for 45 seconds.

Body-Weight Exercises

Alternate Arm/Leg Plank

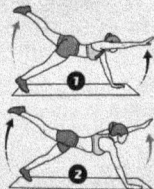

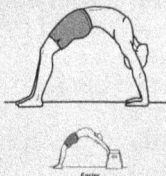

Plank, extend opposite arm and leg, hold.

1. Start in a plank position with hands directly under shoulders.
2. Simultaneously lift and extend your right arm and left leg.
3. Hold this position for a few seconds.
4. Return to the plank position.
5. Repeat with the left arm and right leg.

Army Crawl

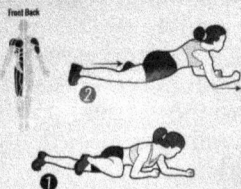

Crawl flat on stomach, using elbows and knees.

1. Lie flat on your stomach with elbows bent and hands directly in front of you.
2. Push with your toes and pull with your elbows to crawl forward.
3. Keep your body low and hips down.
4. Continue crawling for the desired distance or time.

Back Bridge

Plank, extend opposite arm and leg, hold.

1. Lie on your back with knees bent and feet flat on the floor.
2. Place your hands palms down by your sides.
3. Press through your feet and lift your hips up towards the ceiling.
4. Hold this position, squeezing your glutes and keeping your core tight.
5. Lower your hips back down to the starting position.

Bear Crawl

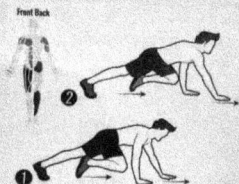

Crawl forward on all fours, hips down, move quickly.

1. Start on all fours with hands under shoulders and knees under hips.
2. Lift your knees slightly off the ground, keeping your back flat.
3. Move your right hand and left foot forward simultaneously.
4. Follow with your left hand and right foot, maintaining a low position.
5. Continue moving forward in this manner quickly.

Bicycle Crunches

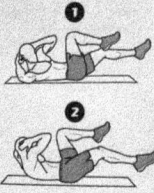

Lie down, alternate elbows to opposite knees cycling legs.

1. Lie on your back with hands behind your head and knees bent.
2. Lift your shoulders off the ground and bring your right elbow towards your left knee while extending the right leg.
3. Switch sides, bringing your left elbow towards your right knee while extending the left leg.
4. Continue alternating sides in a pedaling motion.

Bird Dog

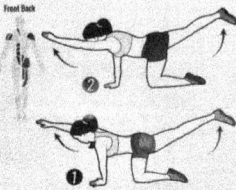

Extend opposite arm and leg, kneeling position.

1. Start on all fours with hands under shoulders and knees under hips.
2. Extend your right arm forward and your left leg backward simultaneously.
3. Hold for a few seconds, keeping your core engaged.
4. Return to the starting position.
5. Repeat with the left arm and right leg.

Bodyweight Row

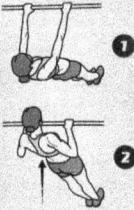

Pull body up towards a bar or table, lying underneath.

1. Position yourself under a bar or table, gripping it with both hands.
2. Keep your body straight and pull your chest up towards the bar.
3. Hold for a moment at the top of the movement.
4. Lower yourself back down to the starting position.
5. Repeat for the desired number of repetitions.

Burpee

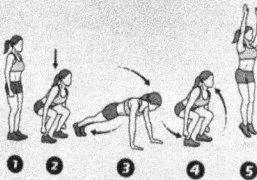

Jump, squat down, kick back into a push-up, return up.

1. Start standing with feet shoulder-width apart.
2. Drop into a squat position and place your hands on the ground.
3. Kick your feet back into a push-up position and lower your body to the ground.
4. Push back up to the push-up position and jump your feet back to your hands.
5. Explosively jump into the air, reaching your arms overhead.
6. Land softly and repeat.

Calf Raise

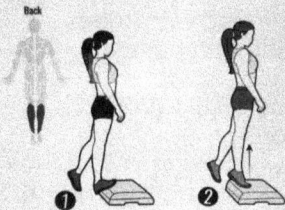

Raise heels off ground, balance on toes, lower slowly.

1. Stand with feet hip-width apart on a flat surface or step.
2. Lift your heels off the ground, balancing on the balls of your feet.
3. Hold the position for a second.
4. Slowly lower your heels back to the ground.
5. Repeat for the desired number of repetitions.

Calf Raises

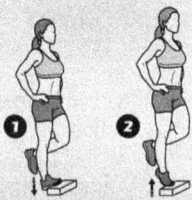

Lift heels off ground, balance on toes, lower slowly.

1. Stand with feet hip-width apart on a flat surface or step.
2. Lift your heels off the ground, balancing on the balls of your feet.
3. Hold the position for a second.
4. Slowly lower your heels back to the ground.
5. Repeat for the desired number of repetitions.

Cat/Camel

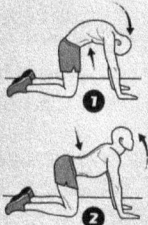

On hands and knees, arch back up and down.

1. Start on all fours with hands under shoulders and knees under hips.
2. Arch your back up towards the ceiling (Cat position).
3. Hold for a few seconds.
4. Lower your back down and lift your head and tailbone up (Camel position).
5. Alternate between the two positions, moving slowly and smoothly.

Crab Toe Touch

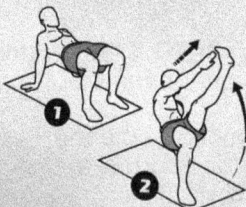

Crawl forward on all fours, hips down, move quickly.

1. Sit on the ground with knees bent, feet flat, and hands behind you.
2. Lift your hips off the ground into a crab position.
3. Reach your right hand to touch your left foot while lifting it.
4. Return to the starting position.
5. Repeat with the left hand and right foot, alternating sides.

Crab Walk

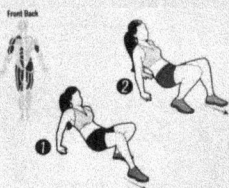

Walk backward on hands and feet, hips elevated.

1. Sit on the ground with knees bent, feet flat, and hands behind you.
2. Lift your hips off the ground into a crab position.
3. Walk backward using your hands and feet, keeping hips elevated.
4. Continue for the desired distance or time.

Crocodile Crawl

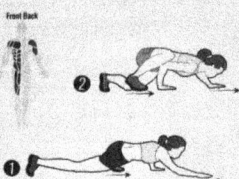

Crawl forward lying almost flat, use elbows and toes.

1. Start in a plank position with elbows bent and body low to the ground.
2. Move forward by simultaneously pulling with one arm and pushing with the opposite leg.
3. Keep your body as low and flat as possible.
4. Continue crawling forward for the desired distance or time.

Cross-Body Crunch

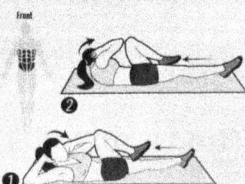

Touch opposite knee to elbow, lying down.

1. Lie on your back with knees bent and hands behind your head.
2. Lift your shoulders off the ground and bring your right elbow towards your left knee while extending the right leg.
3. Return to the starting position.
4. Repeat with the left elbow towards the right knee, alternating sides.

Crunch

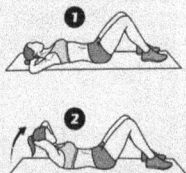

Lift shoulders off ground, contract abdominals.

1. Lie on your back with knees bent and feet flat on the ground.
2. Place your hands behind your head without pulling on your neck.
3. Lift your shoulders off the ground by contracting your abdominal muscles.
4. Hold for a second at the top.
5. Slowly lower back down to the starting position.

Dolphin Kick

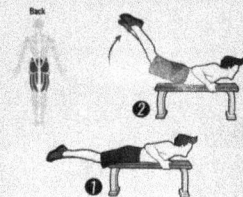

Lie face down, kick legs like a dolphin's tail.

1. Lie face down on a bench with your hips at the edge.
2. Hold onto the bench for support.
3. Lift your legs off the ground, keeping them straight.
4. Kick your legs up and down like a dolphin's tail.
5. Continue for the desired number of repetitions or time.

Donkey Kicks

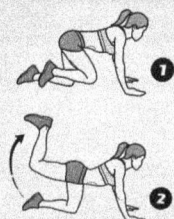

On hands and knees, kick one leg back and up.

1. Start on all fours with hands under shoulders and knees under hips.
2. Keep your right knee bent and lift your right leg up towards the ceiling.
3. Squeeze your glutes at the top.
4. Lower your leg back down without touching the ground.
5. Repeat on the other leg.

Fire Hydrant

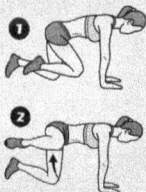

On hands and knees, lift leg to side, keep knee bent.

1. Start on all fours with hands under shoulders and knees under hips.
2. Keep your right knee bent and lift it out to the side.
3. Hold for a moment at the top.
4. Lower your knee back down without touching the ground.
5. Repeat on the other leg.

Flutter Kicks

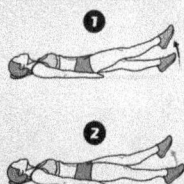

Lie on back, alternately kick legs in small, rapid motion.

1. Lie on your back with hands under your hips for support.
2. Lift both legs off the ground slightly.
3. Alternately kick your legs up and down in a small, rapid motion.
4. Keep your core engaged and back flat on the ground.
5. Continue for the desired time.

Glute Bridge

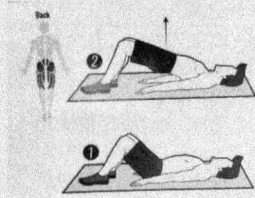

Lift hips while lying on back, feet flat on ground.

1. Lie on your back with knees bent and feet flat on the ground.
2. Place your arms by your sides with palms down.
3. Lift your hips towards the ceiling by squeezing your glutes.
4. Hold for a moment at the top.
5. Lower your hips back to the starting position.

Good Morning

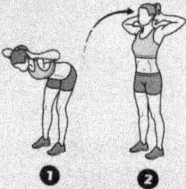

Hinge at hips with hands behind head, focus on hamstrings.

1. Stand with feet shoulder-width apart and hands behind your head.
2. Keep your back straight and hinge at the hips, bending forward.
3. Lower your torso until it's parallel to the ground.
4. Focus on feeling the stretch in your hamstrings.
5. Return to the starting position by engaging your glutes and hamstrings.

Hanging Knee Raise

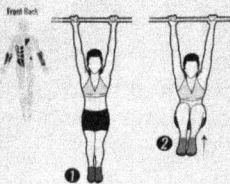

Hang from bar, raise knees towards chest.

1. Hang from a bar with arms extended and feet off the ground.
2. Keep your legs straight and together.
3. Lift your knees towards your chest by engaging your core.
4. Hold for a moment at the top.
5. Lower your legs back to the starting position.

High Knees

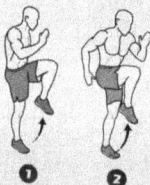

Run in place lifting knees high, maintain pace.

1. Stand with feet hip-width apart.
2. Run in place, lifting your knees as high as possible.
3. Pump your arms in coordination with your legs.
4. Maintain a quick pace and keep your core engaged.
5. Continue for the desired time.

Hip Raise

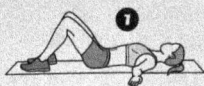

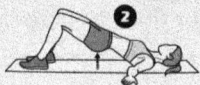

Lift hips while lying on back, feet flat on ground.

1. Lie on your back with knees bent and feet flat on the ground.
2. Place your arms by your sides with palms down.
3. Lift your hips towards the ceiling by squeezing your glutes.
4. Hold for a moment at the top.
5. Lower your hips back to the starting position.
6. Repeat for the desired number of repetitions.

Inchworm

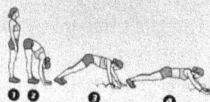

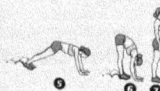

Walk hands forward from standing, hold plank, walk back.

1. Stand with feet hip-width apart.
2. Bend at the waist and place your hands on the ground.
3. Walk your hands forward until you are in a plank position.
4. Hold the plank for a few seconds.
5. Walk your hands back towards your feet and stand up.
6. Repeat for the desired number of repetitions.

Jumping Jacks

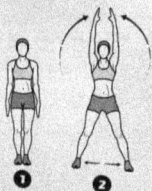

Jump to spread legs and clap hands overhead.

1. Stand with feet together and arms at your sides.
2. Jump to spread your legs while raising your arms overhead to clap.
3. Jump back to the starting position with feet together and arms at your sides.
4. Maintain a quick pace and keep your movements controlled.
5. Repeat for the desired number of repetitions or time.

Leg Pull-In

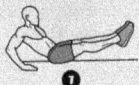

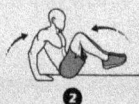

Sit, pull knees into chest, extend legs out.

1. Sit on the ground with legs extended and hands behind you for support.
2. Lean back slightly and lift your legs off the ground.
3. Pull your knees into your chest.
4. Extend your legs back out without touching the ground.
5. Repeat for the desired number of repetitions.

Lunge

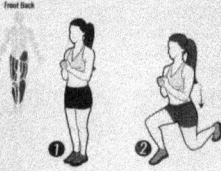

Step forward, lower hips to drop knee to ground.

1. Stand with feet hip-width apart.
2. Step forward with your right leg and lower your hips to drop your right knee towards the ground.
3. Ensure your right knee is directly above your ankle.
4. Push through your right heel to return to the starting position.
5. Repeat with the left leg, alternating sides.

Lying Leg Lift

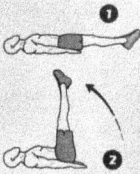

Raise legs vertically, lying flat on back.

1. Lie flat on your back with legs extended and arms by your sides.
2. Keep your legs straight and lift them towards the ceiling until they form a 90-degree angle with your torso.
3. Hold for a moment at the top.
4. Lower your legs back down without touching the ground.
5. Repeat for the desired number of repetitions.

Mountain Climber

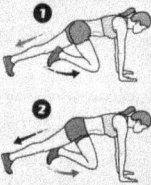

Run in place in plank position, drive knees to chest.

1. Start in a plank position with hands under shoulders and body in a straight line.
2. Bring your right knee towards your chest.
3. Quickly switch legs, bringing your left knee towards your chest while extending your right leg back.
4. Continue alternating legs in a running motion.
5. Maintain a quick pace and keep your core engaged.

Pike Push Up

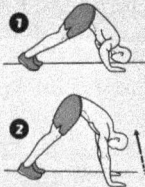

Push-up with hips high, resembles downward dog pose.

1. Start in a downward dog position with hips high and hands shoulder-width apart.
2. Lower your head towards the ground by bending your elbows.
3. Push through your hands to return to the starting position.
4. Keep your body in an inverted V shape throughout the movement.
5. Repeat for the desired number of repetitions.

Plank Rotation

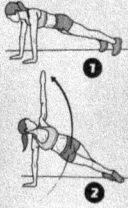

Rotate body in plank, extend arm upward, switch sides.

1. Stand with feet hip-width apart.
2. Step forward with your right leg and lower your hips to drop your right knee towards the ground.
3. Ensure your right knee is directly above your ankle.
4. Push through your right heel to return to the starting position.
5. Repeat with the left leg, alternating sides.

Pull Up

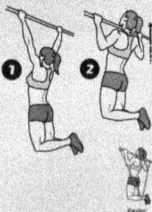

Pull body up on bar, chin above hands.

1. Hang from a pull-up bar with hands shoulder-width apart and palms facing away.
2. Engage your core and pull your body up until your chin is above the bar.
3. Hold for a moment at the top.
4. Lower yourself back down to the starting position with control.
5. Repeat for the desired number of repetitions.

Push Up

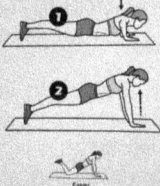

Lower body to ground, push up with arms.

1. Start in a plank position with hands slightly wider than shoulder-width apart.
2. Lower your body towards the ground by bending your elbows.
3. Keep your body in a straight line from head to heels.
4. Push through your hands to return to the starting position.
5. Repeat for the desired number of repetitions.

Push-Back

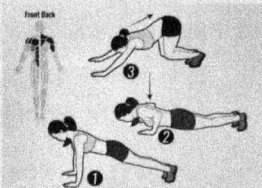

Push body back from push-up position to heels.

1. Start in a plank position with hands under shoulders.
2. Push your hips back towards your heels while keeping your arms extended.
3. Lower your chest towards the ground.
4. Return to the starting plank position.
5. Repeat for the desired number of repetitions.

Push-Up w/ Extension

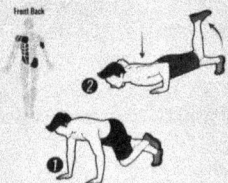

Perform push-up, extend one
arm forward, alternate.

1. Start in a plank position with hands under shoulders.
2. Perform a push-up by lowering your body to the ground.
3. As you push back up, extend your right arm forward.
4. Return your hand to the ground.
5. Repeat with the left arm, alternating sides.

Reverse Crunch

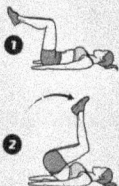

Lift hips off floor, knees
towards chest.

1. Lie on your back with knees bent and feet flat on the ground.
2. Place your hands by your sides or under your hips for support.
3. Lift your hips off the ground and bring your knees towards your chest.
4. Hold for a moment at the top.
5. Lower your hips back to the starting position.
6. Repeat for the desired number of repetitions.

Reverse Plank

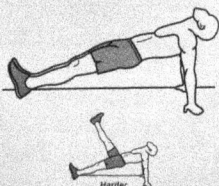

Sit, lift body with arms, legs
straight, face up.

1. Sit on the ground with legs extended and hands behind you, fingers pointing forward.
2. Lift your hips off the ground by pressing through your hands and heels.
3. Keep your body in a straight line from head to heels.
4. Hold for the desired time.
5. Lower your hips back to the ground.

Russian Twist

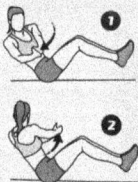

Twist torso holding weight,
seated on ground.

1. Sit on the ground with knees bent and feet flat.
2. Lean back slightly and lift your feet off the ground, balancing on your sit bones.
3. Hold a weight with both hands and twist your torso to the right, bringing the weight beside your hip.
4. Twist to the left, bringing the weight to the other side.
5. Continue alternating sides for the desired number of repetitions.

Scissor Kick

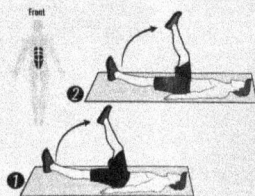

Alternately lift legs in lying position, engages core.

1. Lie flat on your back with hands under your hips for support.
2. Lift your legs slightly off the ground.
3. Alternately lift one leg higher while lowering the other leg, keeping both legs straight.
4. Continue the scissor motion, engaging your core throughout.
5. Repeat for the desired number of repetitions or time.

Side Crunches

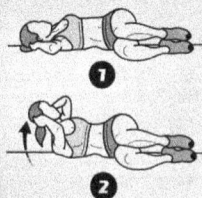

Lie on side, perform crunches towards elevated leg.

1. Lie on your side with legs bent and hands behind your head.
2. Lift your upper body towards your hips, crunching towards the elevated leg.
3. Squeeze your obliques at the top of the movement.
4. Lower back down to the starting position.
5. Repeat for the desired number of repetitions, then switch sides.

Side Lunge

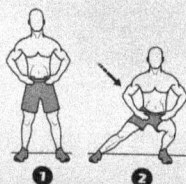

Step to side into lunge, keep other leg straight.

1. Stand with feet hip-width apart.
2. Step to the side with your right leg, lowering your hips into a lunge.
3. Keep your left leg straight and your chest up.
4. Push through your right foot to return to the starting position.
5. Repeat on the other side, alternating legs.

Side Plank

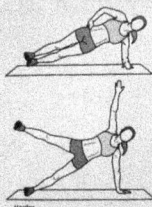

Support body on one arm, side facing ground.

1. Lie on your side with your elbow directly under your shoulder.
2. Lift your hips off the ground, forming a straight line from head to feet.
3. Hold this position, keeping your core engaged.
4. For added difficulty, extend your top arm towards the ceiling.
5. Repeat on the other side.

Side-to-Side Pull-Up

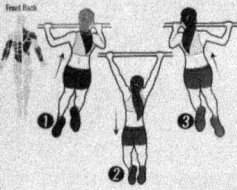

Pull up and move sideways along bar, alternate sides.

1. Hang from a pull-up bar with hands shoulder-width apart.
2. Pull your body up towards the bar, moving to the right side.
3. Lower yourself back down and pull up again, moving to the left side.
4. Continue alternating sides.
5. Repeat for the desired number of repetitions.

Side-to-Side Push-Up

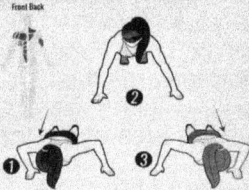

Shift side-to-side during push-ups, engages core.

1. Start in a plank position with hands slightly wider than shoulder-width apart.
2. Lower your body towards the ground, shifting your weight to the right.
3. Push back up and shift your weight to the left.
4. Continue alternating sides with each push-up.
5. Repeat for the desired number of repetitions.

Single Leg Dead Lift

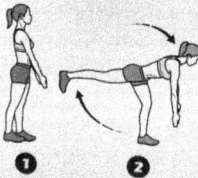

Balance on one leg, hinge forward, extend free leg back.

1. Stand on your right leg with a slight bend in the knee.
2. Hinge at the hips, extending your left leg back and lowering your torso towards the ground.
3. Keep your back straight and core engaged.
4. Return to the starting position by squeezing your glutes.
5. Repeat on the other leg, alternating sides.

Single Leg Split Squat

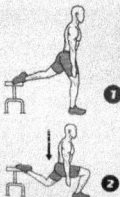

Perform split squat on one leg, elevated rear foot.

1. Stand a few feet in front of a bench or elevated surface.
2. Place your right foot behind you on the bench.
3. Lower your hips into a squat, keeping your left knee over your ankle.
4. Push through your left heel to return to the starting position.
5. Repeat on the other leg, alternating sides.

Single Leg Squat

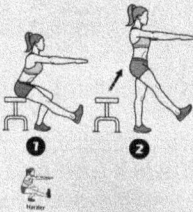

Stand on one leg, squat, maintain balance.

1. Stand on your right leg, extending your left leg in front.
2. Lower your hips into a squat, keeping your left leg elevated.
3. Maintain balance and keep your chest up.
4. Push through your right heel to return to the starting position.
5. Repeat on the other leg, alternating sides.

Skater Squat

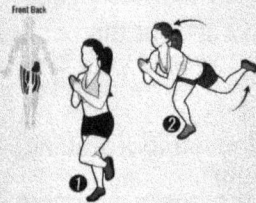

Balance on one leg, squat, touch opposite hand to foot.

1. Balance on your right leg, bending your left knee.
2. Lower into a squat while reaching your left hand towards your right foot.
3. Keep your back straight and chest up.
4. Push through your right heel to return to the starting position.
5. Repeat on the other leg, alternating sides.

Spiderman

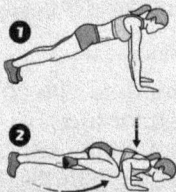

Bring knee to elbow during push-up, switch sides.

1. Start in a push-up position with hands under shoulders.
2. Lower your body towards the ground while bringing your right knee to your right elbow.
3. Push back up to the starting position.
4. Repeat with the left knee to the left elbow, alternating sides.
5. Continue for the desired number of repetitions.

Squat

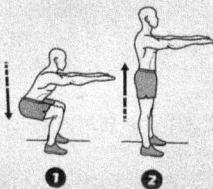

Stand, bend knees to lower body, keep back straight.

1. Stand with feet shoulder-width apart and arms extended in front.
2. Bend your knees and lower your hips into a squat.
3. Keep your back straight and chest up.
4. Push through your heels to return to the starting position.
5. Repeat for the desired number of repetitions.

Star Plank

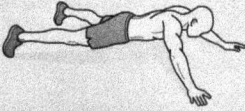

Extend arms and legs out from body in plank position.

1. Start in a plank position with hands under shoulders and feet together.
2. Extend your right arm and left leg out to the sides.
3. Hold for a moment, keeping your core engaged.
4. Return to the starting position and repeat with the left arm and right leg.
5. Alternate sides for the desired number of repetitions.

Step Up

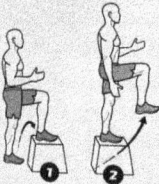

Step onto a raised platform, alternate legs.

1. Stand in front of a raised platform or bench.
2. Step up with your right foot, bringing your left knee towards your chest.
3. Step back down with your left foot, then your right foot.
4. Repeat with the left foot leading, alternating sides.
5. Continue for the desired number of repetitions.

Stretching

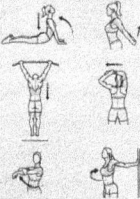

Perform various stretches to improve flexibility and cool down.

1. Perform a variety of stretches, targeting all major muscle groups.
2. Hold each stretch for 15-30 seconds.
3. Focus on slow, controlled movements to increase flexibility.
4. Include stretches for the hamstrings, quadriceps, calves, chest, back, and shoulders.
5. Ensure a thorough cool-down to aid in recovery.

Sumo Squat

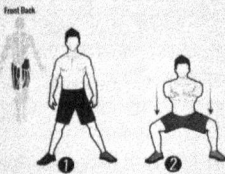

Wide stance squat, toes pointed out, lower body.

1. Stand with feet wider than shoulder-width apart and toes pointed out.
2. Lower your hips into a squat, keeping your back straight and chest up.
3. Ensure your knees track over your toes.
4. Push through your heels to return to the starting position.
5. Repeat for the desired number of repetitions.

Superman

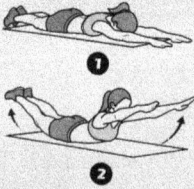

Extend arms and legs while face down, hold position.

1. Lie face down on the ground with arms extended forward and legs straight.
2. Lift your arms, chest, and legs off the ground simultaneously.
3. Hold the top position for a few seconds.
4. Lower back down to the starting position.
5. Repeat for the desired number of repetitions.

Swimmer

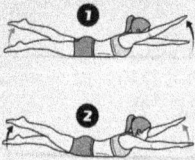

Lie face down, alternate lifting arms and legs.

1. Lie face down on the ground with arms extended forward and legs straight.
2. Lift your right arm and left leg off the ground simultaneously.
3. Lower them back down and lift your left arm and right leg.
4. Continue alternating sides in a swimming motion.
5. Repeat for the desired number of repetitions or time.

Tricep Dip

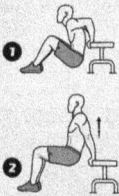

Dip body between bars, focus on triceps.

1. Sit on the edge of a bench or chair with hands gripping the edge.
2. Slide your hips off the edge, supporting your weight with your arms.
3. Lower your body by bending your elbows to a 90-degree angle.
4. Push through your palms to return to the starting position.
5. Repeat for the desired number of repetitions.

Tricep Push Up

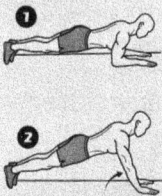

Push-up with hands under shoulders, elbows tight.

1. Start in a plank position with hands under shoulders and elbows close to your body.
2. Lower your body towards the ground, keeping elbows tight to your sides.
3. Push through your palms to return to the starting position.
4. Keep your body in a straight line throughout the movement.
5. Repeat for the desired number of repetitions.

Tuck Jumps

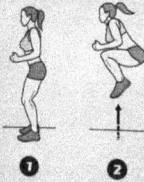

Jump high, tuck knees to chest mid-air.

1. Stand with feet hip-width apart and knees slightly bent.
2. Jump explosively, bringing your knees towards your chest.
3. Land softly on the balls of your feet with knees slightly bent.
4. Immediately jump again, maintaining quick, controlled movements.
5. Repeat for the desired number of repetitions or time.

V Up

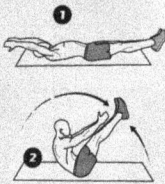

Lie back, lift legs and torso simultaneously, form 'V'.

1. Lie on your back with arms extended overhead and legs straight.
2. Simultaneously lift your legs and torso off the ground, reaching your hands towards your feet.
3. Form a "V" shape with your body at the top of the movement.
4. Lower back down to the starting position with control.
5. Repeat for the desired number of repetitions.

Walking Lunge

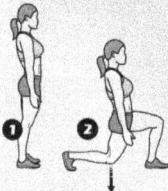

Step forward into a lunge, move forward alternating legs.

1. Stand with feet hip-width apart and hands on your hips.
2. Step forward with your right leg, lowering into a lunge.
3. Push through your right heel to stand and bring your left leg forward into the next lunge.
4. Continue alternating legs, moving forward with each step.
5. Repeat for the desired number of repetitions or distance.

Walking Toe Touches

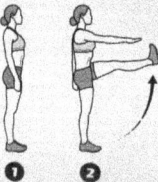

Walk, reach down to touch toes with opposite hand.

1. Stand with feet hip-width apart.
2. Step forward with your right leg, lifting it straight in front of you.
3. Reach your left hand to touch your right toes.
4. Lower your leg and step forward with your left leg, reaching your right hand to your left toes.
5. Continue alternating sides as you walk forward.

Wall Sit

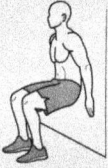

Sit against wall, legs at 90 degrees, hold position.

1. Stand with your back against a wall.
2. Slide down the wall until your thighs are parallel to the ground.
3. Keep your feet shoulder-width apart and knees at a 90-degree angle.
4. Hold this position for the desired amount of time.
5. Maintain tension in your thighs and keep your back flat against the wall.

Wall Squat

Front Back

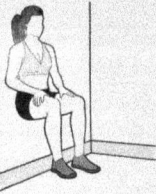

Lie face down, alternate lifting arms and legs.

1. Stand with your back against a wall, feet shoulder-width apart.
2. Slide down into a squat position, keeping your back against the wall.
3. Ensure your thighs are parallel to the ground and knees are above your ankles.
4. Hold this position for the desired time.
5. Maintain proper form by keeping your back straight and core engaged.

Wide/Narrow Push Up

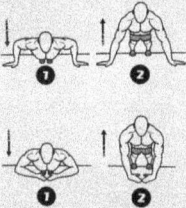

Perform push-ups with varying hand widths.

1. Start in a plank position with hands wider than shoulder-width apart.
2. Lower your body to the ground by bending your elbows.
3. Push through your palms to return to the starting position.
4. Move your hands closer together, directly under your shoulders.
5. Perform another push-up in this narrow position.
6. Alternate between wide and narrow push-ups for the desired repetitions.

Windshield Wiper

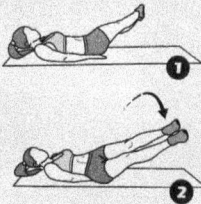

Swing legs side-to-side lying down, mimic wiper.

1. Lie on your back with arms extended out to the sides for support.
2. Lift your legs off the ground and bring them to a 90-degree angle.
3. Slowly lower your legs to the right side, keeping them together.
4. Bring your legs back to the center.
5. Lower your legs to the left side.
6. Continue alternating sides, mimicking a windshield wiper motion.

www.ingramcontent.com/pod-product-compliance
Lightning Source LLC
Chambersburg PA
CBHW031549260326
41914CB00002B/336